EFFECTIVE
COMMUNICATION
for Nursing Associates

Sara Miller McCune founded SAGE Publishing in 1965 to support the dissemination of usable knowledge and educate a global community. SAGE publishes more than 1000 journals and over 800 new books each year, spanning a wide range of subject areas. Our growing selection of library products includes archives, data, case studies and video. SAGE remains majority owned by our founder and after her lifetime will become owned by a charitable trust that secures the company's continued independence.

Los Angeles | London | New Delhi | Singapore | Washington DC | Melbourne

KERRY WELCH

EFFECTIVE
COMMUNICATION
for Nursing Associates

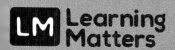
LM Learning Matters

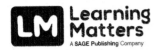

Learning Matters
A SAGE Publishing Company
1 Oliver's Yard
55 City Road
London EC1Y 1SP

SAGE Publications Inc.
2455 Teller Road
Thousand Oaks, California 91320

SAGE Publications India Pvt Ltd
B 1/I 1 Mohan Cooperative Industrial Area
Mathura Road
New Delhi 110 044

SAGE Publications Asia-Pacific Pte Ltd
3 Church Street
#10-04 Samsung Hub
Singapore 049483

Editor: Laura Walmsley
Development editor: Eleanor Rivers
Senior project editor: Chris Marke
Project management: River Editorial
Marketing manager: Ruslana Khatagova
Cover design: Wendy Scott
Typeset by: C&M Digitals (P) Ltd, Chennai, India
Printed in the UK

Library of Congress Control Number: 2022930444

British Library Cataloguing in Publication Data

A catalogue record for this book is available from
the British Library

ISBN 978-1-5297-5476-6
ISBN 978-1-5297-5475-9 (pbk)

At SAGE we take sustainability seriously. Most of our products are printed in the UK using responsibly sourced
papers and boards. When we print overseas we ensure sustainable papers are used as measured by the
PREPS grading system. We undertake an annual audit to monitor our sustainability.

Contents

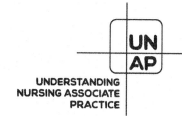

UNDERSTANDING NURSING ASSOCIATE PRACTICE

Supporting you through your nursing associate training & career

UNDERSTANDING NURSING ASSOCIATE PRACTICE is a series uniquely designed for trainee nursing associates.

Each book in the series is:

- Mapped to the NMC standards of proficiency for nursing associates
- Affordable
- Full of practical activities & case studies
- Focused on clearly explaining theory & its application to practice

Current books in the series include:

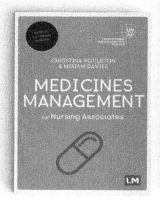
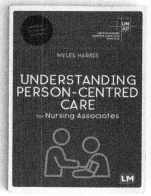
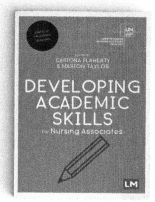

Visit
uk.sagepub.com/UNAP
for more information

About the author

Kerry Welch has been a registered nurse since 1995 and has worked in a wide variety of clinical settings and environments. This includes in intensive care (neurological and general), then latterly in primary care as a Practice Nurse. Kerry has an in-flight nursing award and qualifications in both intensive care and primary care, as well as an MSc in Medical Ethics. The MSc drove her interest in nurse education, and she has been a lecturer and senior lecturer in higher education since 2006. Kerry has a teaching qualification which is recorded with the NMC and is the lead for the Nursing Associate programme at the University of Lincoln. She is passionate about the role of the nursing associate in healthcare and is proud to have been involved in the training of nursing associates since 2018.

Acknowledgements

Writing this book during a pandemic has had its challenges, so I would like to thank the supportive team at SAGE Publishing for their valuable input into the book's development.

I would like to thank my husband Dan and our children Lucy and Oliver for listening to me mumble about chapter content, for their encouragement and for giving me additional time to write.

I would also like to acknowledge Mandie Riggs, for her unfaltering belief in me, and Mr Sherman the eight-year-old Staffy-cross rescue pup, for his companionship.

Kerry Welch
January 2022

Introduction

Who is this book for?

This book is specifically aimed at trainee and registered nursing associates. This book also has many transferable elements and content which would make it relevant for all current and aspiring healthcare and social care workers, or those interested in understanding communication and the practical application of communication skills.

About the book

The purpose of this book started out as a general introduction to communication in healthcare, specifically aimed at meeting the Nursing and Midwifery Council *Standards and Proficiencies for Registered Nursing Associates* (2018c). The book quickly evolved into a practical road map of communication in health and social care settings, with a solid underpinning of theory.

The book explores many of the challenges of communicating with patients, particularly when giving technical or upsetting information. It looks at team working and development towards leadership and being a role model, giving the reader opportunities to develop awareness of those communication challenges and how to address them in both a professional and practical manner while meeting the NMC standards.

All the content within this book is designed to enable you to deliver safe, effective and meaningful care to patients and their loved ones as a professional nursing associate. This book also encourages the reader to engage in a wide variety of activities which puts communication at the heart of professional awareness, understanding and personal development, to make you the best nursing associate you can be.

Book structure

Chapter 1. The theory behind effective communication

This chapter starts by introducing communication as a fundamental element of high-quality, person-centred nursing practice. It includes a general exploration of communication, how communication theory has developed and what it means in practice. The various methods of communication are explored and how these methods can influence the patient's role as an active participant in their care is discussed.

Chapter 2. Professional communication

In this chapter, the variety of ways in which information is shared, delivered or interpreted is explored. With a consideration of how to share information, this chapter includes case studies to illustrate how giving information, using correct telephone etiquette, verbal handovers and maintaining confidentiality can be applied in practice.

Chapter 3. Interpersonal relationships

This chapter links with Chapter 9 and looks at how the individual can start building relationships that will enable them to develop their professional identity as a nursing associate and find their place in a team.

The chapter covers behaviours, skills and attitudes, as well as the 6Cs, which are care, compassion, courage, communication, commitment and competence (NHS England, 2012). Activities facilitate self-awareness and an understanding of how nursing associates respond to others, at all levels of healthcare provision. Interprofessional working and collaboration with the multidisciplinary team is the focus throughout.

Chapter 4. Communication in diverse settings

One of the factors that makes the role of the nursing associate unique is that it is a generalist qualification covering all four fields of nursing. Once registered, nursing associates will be able to care for all patients wherever care is delivered. This chapter outlines the various factors that need to be considered for communication to be effective and appropriate, regardless of the care setting.

Chapter 5. Challenges to effective communication in clinical practice

The ability to communicate effectively with sensitivity and compassion is an essential skill for all healthcare professionals. This chapter explores the challenges heightened emotions can bring to communication for the practitioner, the patient, families and their carers, and how these can be addressed. Challenging situations, such as anger, death, dying, bereavement and loss, can result in difficult conversations in practice. The chapter equips nursing associates with the ability to translate the theory into empathic practice to better understand patients and their own role in such situations.

Chapter 6. Inclusive communication

This chapter outlines some of the terminology and legislation surrounding diversity and equality. It outlines the protected characteristics as included in the 2010 Equality Act (HMSO, 2010) and explores what discrimination can look like in practice. The chapter introduces and helps the reader to engage with inclusive language. It also explores bias in order to help the reader better recognise and challenge it.

Chapter 7. Communicating with patients who have specialist requirements

This chapter contains guidance on how to communicate with children or adults who have a specific diagnosis or learning difficulty that may need reasonable adjustments to accommodate them while receiving care. The chapter explores sensory deficits including hearing, sight and speech that can affect many people across the lifespan and will influence their ability to access and receive care.

Chapter 8. Assessment and support in clinical practice for the nursing associate role

Once qualified, a nursing associate will be expected to undertake supervision of others in practice. Case studies and learning activities within this chapter are used to show how effective decision making and constructive feedback can become positive 'teachable moments'. Moreover, how motivational questioning and specific communication techniques can enhance the therapeutic relationship for student, patient and carer.

Chapter 9. Finding your own voice

This final chapter consolidates knowledge from theory, the previous chapters and practice experiences. It assists the reader to learn about themselves in order to define their own personal professional identity. The expected goal is for the reader to demonstrate that professional boundaries have been learned allowing integrity, autonomy and leadership styles to flourish in a rapidly changing healthcare workforce.

Requirements for the NMC Future Nurse Standards of Proficiency for Nursing Associates

The Nursing and Midwifery Council (NMC) has established standards of proficiency to be met by applicants to different parts of the register, and these are the standards it considers necessary for safe and effective practice. This book is structured so that it will help you to understand and meet the proficiencies required for entry to the NMC register as a nursing associate. The relevant proficiencies are presented at the start of each chapter so that you can clearly see which ones the chapter addresses. The proficiencies have been designed to be generic so apply to all fields of nursing and all care settings. This is because all nursing associates must be able to meet the needs of any person they encounter in their practice, regardless of the person's stage of life or health challenges, and whether these are mental, physical, cognitive or behavioural.

This book includes the latest standards for 2018 onwards, taken from the *Standards of Proficiency for Nursing Associates* (NMC, 2018c).

Learning features

Textbooks can be intimidating and learning from reading text is not always easy. However, this series has been designed specifically to help the nursing associate learn from the books within it. By using a number of learning features throughout the books, they will help you to develop your understanding and ability to apply theory to practice, while remaining engaging and breaking the text up into manageable chunks. This book contains activities, case studies, theory summary boxes, further reading, useful websites and other materials to enable you to participate in your own learning. The book cannot provide all the answers, but it provides a good outline of the most important information and helps you build a framework for your own learning.

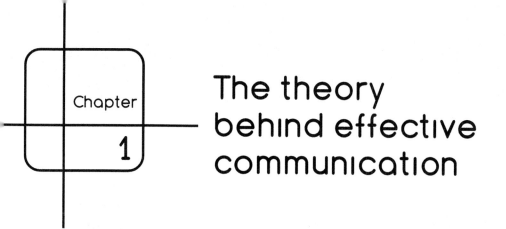

The theory behind effective communication

Chapter 1

NMC FUTURE NURSE STANDARDS OF PROFICIENCY FOR NURSING ASSOCIATES

This chapter will address the following platforms and proficiencies:

Platform 1: Being an accountable professional

At the point of registration, the nursing associate will be able to:

1.9   communicate effectively using a range of skills and strategies with colleagues and people at all stages of life and with a range of mental, physical, cognitive and behavioural health challenges.

Annexe A: Communication and relationship management skills

At the point of registration, the nursing associate will be able to safely demonstrate the following skills:

1.   Underpinning communication skills for providing and monitoring care:
1.1   actively listen, recognise and respond to verbal and non-verbal cues.
1.2   use prompts and positive verbal and non-verbal reinforcement.
1.3   use appropriate non-verbal communication including touch, eye contact and personal space.
1.4   make appropriate use of open and closed questioning.
1.5   speak clearly and accurately.
1.6   use caring conversation techniques.
1.7   check understanding and use clarification techniques.
1.12   recognise the need for translator services and material.
1.13   use age-appropriate communication techniques.

> ## Chapter aims
>
> By the end of this chapter, you will be able to:
>
> - define what communication is.
> - discuss different types of communication.
> - describe the development of communication theory.
> - identify some models of communication and their relevance to the nursing associate role.
> - explore how we communicate.

Introduction

This chapter begins by defining communication and then introducing the four main types of communication. The focus is on non-verbal communication to help you learn how to be an active observer, as a key developmental step in becoming an effective nursing associate. Being able to look for, correctly identify and filter the messages from the grandiose to the minute allows us to explore communication and its uses. Finally, the chapter presents key models of communication, an understanding of which will help you combine your nursing skills with communication tools to enhance your therapeutic relationship with those in your care.

Definition

Take a moment to look around your current surroundings. I think it would be fair to say that communication is everywhere, one for the fact you are holding this book and reading this sentence, or having the sentence read to you. Communication bombards us from the noises around you and the signs and symbols that adorn our lives, which direct us and help us negotiate the environment. If you are a driver, think about how long you took to learn the road signs for your driving test and how they help you navigate the road networks. If you walk, traffic lights help us know where it is safe to cross the road.

Despite the prevalence of communication surrounding us, communication itself is difficult to define. Individuals will define communication in a way which is relevant to their interests and their perspective. If you were interested in technology and computing, you may refer to it as an interface, which is a device or programme which allows a user to communicate with a computer.

The word 'communication' comes from the Latin word *communis*, which means 'common'. So 'to communicate' means 'to make common' or 'to make known', 'to share', and includes all forms of what we would call communication, so verbal, non-verbal and electronic means of human interaction (Velentzas and Broni, 2014).

A dictionary definition would be, simply, that communication is a process of imparting or exchanging information between individuals through a common system of symbols, signs or behaviour.

One other definition of communication is given to us by Mehrabian (1972, p. 2) who states that:

> Any act by which one person gives to or receives from another person information about that person's needs, desires, perceptions, knowledge, or affective states. Communication may be intentional or unintentional, may involve conventional or unconventional signals, may take linguistic or non-linguistic forms, and may occur through spoken or other modes.

Mehrabian's definition is very thorough, as it includes both expressed communication and the involuntary or accidental communication. An awareness that communication takes many forms and can be intentional or unintentional is important for your role as a nursing associate because you will be communicating with a wide range of individuals from a vast variety of backgrounds and levels of education and experience. This knowledge will help you adapt your communication to reflect the needs of the person you are communicating with.

What we communicate

Communication is a fundamental aspect of human existence and survival: it gives us the means to express our common goals and it identifies us as unique individuals. It helps keep us and others safe from harm and allows us to experience a vast array of emotions.

Outward expression, as a means of communication, is essential for engaging with others, but if we choose not to engage with others, we cannot just turn communication 'off'. Our bodies continue to communicate through actions and reactions even if we don't want to communicate anything.

Every movement, whether purposeful or through a spontaneous reaction to stimuli, betrays our thoughts, feelings and intentions to the active observer. Purely reactive communication doesn't require any thought. If someone were to encounter an odour that they considered bad or offensive, they would naturally wrinkle or cover their nose. This reaction does not require thought or decision but is courtesy of the autonomic nervous system engaging with internal protective mechanisms.

An observer would interpret physical actions automatically and would know that there was a bad odour that was best avoided. Here is where our similarity to the animal kingdom can be seen most keenly. Activity 1.1 explores these similarities in more depth.

Activity 1.1 Critical thinking

This activity is asking you to use your lived experiences to explore the common aspects of communication between animals and humans.

As an observer in a busy town centre, you see a family sitting on a bench feeding the birds. They have managed to attract the attention of approximately 30 birds, who are bustling around each other, hungrily pecking at the bird food from the pavement. What do you expect would happen if there was a sudden, unexpected loud noise from behind the busy pigeons and in front of the family? Why?

An outline answer is provided at the end of the chapter.

From Activity 1.1, we can see that communication is essential to our being, but we often fail to effectively communicate, which leads to misinterpretation of the messages being received. If communication were effective, we should never leave an encounter with feelings of confusion or frustration. The fact that those feelings are commonplace in everyday life highlights the importance of getting communication right in a healthcare setting. Having a patient left confused about their care or frustrated by what is happening to them is wholly unsatisfactory.

It is little wonder that communication in its many forms has been a subject for study for many years. Most notably, communication theory developed with the increasing use of information technology in the 1920s.

Whatever type of communication is used, we need the same basic elements for communication to occur. We need some form of sender or delivery system, a message or information to send and an audience for the information or recipient. For the communication to be clear, the sender and the receiver must share some similarities, such as a common language. Activity 1.2 encourages you to think about how to communicate.

Methods of communication

Activity 1.2   Reflection

This activity asks you to consider all the possible ways in which we communicate. Before reading on, write down all the possible ways in which we communicate that you can think of.

An outline answer is provided at the end of the chapter.

Activity 1.2 has introduced you to the variety of ways in which we communicate. We use communication every day in nearly every environment. Whether you give a slight head nod in agreement, momentarily frown, or present information to a large group, communication is necessary.

Learning and developing good communication skills can help you improve as a care giver and a valuable team member. While it takes time and practice, communication and interpersonal skills can be developed and refined.

From your work in Activity 1.2, you will have realised that there are four main methods of communication: verbal, non-verbal, written and visual.

Verbal communication

When most people think about communication, they tend to think of spoken language first. Verbal communication includes those methods of communication such as spoken language and sign language, as well as laughter and crying. Verbal communication is a quick and efficient means to get a point across. It is best used in conjunction with another of the methods, such as non-verbal and written. Verbal communication is often supported by paraverbal or paralinguistic communication, which is expressed through grunting sounds but also by the tone, speed and volume of the communication (Kjellmer, 2009).

Once you have established what you want to communicate and have decided that verbal communication is the best way, it is important also to consider how to engage the words and the voice to give the message the desired emphasis. Things to consider include:

Voice tone: This refers to *how* you say something rather than what is said. I have no doubt many of us have been scolded with 'Don't talk to me in that tone of voice!'

Voice speed: Talking quickly can convey agitation or excitement. It can leave people feeling bemused and confused. It is important that you pace your speech so that the listener can keep up.

Voice volume: This ranges from an inaudible whisper to shouting and screaming and anything between. Obviously, people being able to hear you while attempting to communicate verbally would be a prerequisite for communication being effective. Likewise, shouting test results to a patient in a busy clinic is inappropriate.

The language used: Consider whether the patient understands the language you are using. Think about alternatives to ensure that you are giving as much information as they need to be able to understand; this may be by keeping the words simple or the use of a translator who is not a family member.

Vocabulary used: Medicine is littered with long Latin words and complex names for procedures and medicines, as well as frequent abbreviations, **acronyms** and symbols. This can result in people easily getting lost in the language. Activity 1.3 challenges your understanding of some commonly used medical language abbreviations and shortcuts.

Activity 1.3   Work-based learning

In healthcare, there are a huge number of medical abbreviations and shortcuts that are in common use. Can you decode some of those seen in Figure 1.1?

IM		EEG		Stat	
TPR		ECG		#	
BNO		QDS		CXR	
NBM		PRN		DNAR	

Figure 1.1 Common medical abbreviations.

The answers are provided at the end of the chapter.

Having completed Activity 1.3, you will see that medical communication can be complex and confusing, but, as with anything that you practise enough, it will become second nature. With vocabulary, we also need to be cautious about the use of slang terms and colloquialisms that are regionally or culturally specific, as this could lead to confusion and cause offence. Similarly, the use of swearing and general curse words is not recommended for a professional nursing associate.

The use of grammar: Grammar is defined as the set of structural rules that govern the composition of sentences, phrases and words in language. Using correct grammar to organise your speech helps you make the right emphasis on what is being said. An example of poor grammar might be 'She gave the medicine to the patient in the refrigerator', as opposed to 'She gave the medicine in the refrigerator to the patient'. As you can see, poor grammar can significantly alter the meaning of a sentence, so it is important to get this right.

Non-verbal communication

Non-verbal communication is useful when we are trying to understand what people think or feel. Non-verbal expressions range from subtle, unintentional movement such as raising an eyebrow, to a full-on, intentional bear hug, and so much more between.

Being able to 'read' non-verbal language is a skill we possess from birth. It is more universal than any spoken language and equates to around 70–90% of all our communication (Mehrabian, 1972). The more people we meet, the more we develop the skill of reading the physical behaviour of the body. There is no place where this is more important than when helping people who are anxious, scared or angry; often, patients are in these states when they meet us, and we need to learn how to recognise those feelings and be able to address them.

Non-verbal communication is typically a whole-body affair. Starting at the top, we explore the role the head has in non-verbal communication.

The head

The head alone can convey a series of emotions and feelings, which can have a cultural significance. In the UK, we tend to accept that a nod of the head is a positive 'yes' statement while a shake of the head is a negative 'no' statement. If we are effectively listening, if we agree or disagree with what is being said, we will nod or shake our heads as a means of expression. These movements are often associated with paraverbal or paralinguistic 'backchannels', such as the use of 'Umm...Hmmm...Uh huh' (Kjellmer, 2009).

However, we need to be mindful that nodding the head to mean 'yes' is not a universally accepted behaviour. In countries such as Bulgaria and Greece, nodding means 'no'. Shaking the head from side to side in South Asian culture may mean, 'yes', 'good', 'okay', 'I understand' or 'maybe', depending on the nature of the conversation (Axtell, 1998). A tilted head requires a little more information from facial expressions to communicate the meaning. A tilted head could be 'I'm thinking' or 'I'm confused'.

Facial expressions

Facial expressions are arguably the most common mechanism for non-verbal expression and the one area we endeavour to control. The social learning and cultural emphasis on controlling facial expressions is significant (Frank, 2001). The British are renowned for their 'stiff upper lip'; similarly, in Japanese culture, it is desirable to demonstrate the characteristic of self-control.

There are seven basic emotions expressed on the face as a single expression of emotion. A single expression or **macroexpression** of emotion will appear on the face for a duration of between 0.5 and 4 seconds and involve the whole face (Ekman, 2003). These macroexpressions occur with a single emotion and are difficult to modify or conceal. They occur when we are alone and when we are with people whom we consider close to us.

Another important aspect of facial expressions are **microexpressions**. Microexpressions are expressions which appear on the face and are gone again in a matter of fractions of a second and are most likely caused by concealed emotions and possible deception (Ekman, 2003). An interesting factor in facial expressions is the difference between a genuine and fake smile. The Duchenne smile, as described by the French neurologist Guillaume Duchenne in the early nineteenth century, characterises a genuine smile which comes from an expression of true enjoyment (Beamish et al., 2019). A genuine smile involves the use of the zygomaticus major muscle, which lifts the corners of the mouth. At the same time, the orbicularis oculi muscles lift your cheeks and crinkle your eyes at the corners. We identify a fake or false smile by the limited engagement of the orbicularis oculi muscle. If there is no wrinkling around the eyes when there is a broad smile on the face, the smile is a fake one.

It is generally accepted that there are seven universal emotions expressed on the face (Matsumoto et al., 2011):

- joy;
- surprise;
- contempt;
- sadness;
- anger;
- disgust;
- fear.

Eye gaze

It has been said that 'The eyes are the window to the soul', and we can associate other common phrases specific to the gaze: 'Don't look at me like that!'; 'It's rude to stare'; 'I'm watching you!'

Not surprisingly, eye contact and gaze are very important when we communicate, but this process is far from universal. People from Europe, North America, Korea, Thailand and Saudi Arabia regard a direct gaze as behaviour indicating openness and honesty. Individuals from Japan, South America, West Africa and Puerto Rico, however, find direct eye contact to be rude and suggestive of dishonesty (Morris, 2002). Clearly there is a potential to cause offence if you get this wrong.

Establishing eye contact, certainly within the UK, means that we are going to communicate, and it builds a connection. Have you ever tried getting eye contact with a waiter, only for them to look through you because they are busy and don't have time for you right now?

Eye contact within healthcare settings remains a powerful tool. It is a means of developing trust because eye contact indicates an openness to communicate, but also that you are listening. Maintaining eye contact during a conversation shows that you are focused, paying attention and actively listening.

Gestures

Gestures are essentially a non-verbal shorthand, using the movement of body parts, but, most noticeably, the movement of the hands and arms, such as a handshake. The handshake is classed as a relic gesture, which refers to the age of the gesture. Handshakes date back to the fifth century B.C. in Greece, where it was seen as a symbol of peace. The open hand showed that neither person was carrying a weapon. Gestures are a powerful form of communication, which is highlighted in some iconic images and pictures. For example, the raised closed fist has become a symbol of the Black Lives Matter movement. Another enduring example is Winston Churchill's 'V' sign for victory at the end of the Second World War.

With most forms of communication, there is a cultural significance, the thumbs-up sign, for example, is a widely recognised sign of approval or agreement in the UK; however, in Bangladesh, this is an insult, and, in some parts of the Middle East, a thumbs-up is highly offensive (Axtell, 1998).

There are, however, some universal gestures, such as mimic gestures, which are acted-out real actions or objects. Imagine how you would ask your friend if they wanted a drink from across a busy and noisy cafe.

Gesture, as an expression of emotion or thought, is a valuable means of communication, not to be confused with gesticulation, which is to dramatise what is being said and is often demonstrated by individuals who 'talk with their hands'. There are other ways in which we talk with our hands by using coded gestures, such as when using Makaton or sign language.

Body movement and posture

Body movement is the physical expression of our thoughts. As with facial expressions, these movements are difficult, if not impossible, to hide. Posture relates to the stance and height or the 'erectness' of the body. Someone who is standing upright with their shoulders back and their head up would be seen as confident or energised. A stiffness to the body in this state could, however, also be interpreted as aggressive. A stooped posture would be one where the individual is stooped over with their shoulders rolled forward and their head down.

When discussing posture, there is often a reference made to individuals having either an 'open' or 'closed' posture, which reflects the individual's sense of security or confidence and their openness or receptiveness for communication.

Closed posture

A closed posture is indicated by the body being in a 'closed off' position, with either their arms folded in front of them, and/or their legs crossed. They can also tilt the body in a direction away from the person trying to communicate with them. This often indicates that the person is scared, uncomfortable or just not interested.

Open posture

An open posture is characterised by the individual exposing their abdomen and chest with their arms by their side and their legs and feet uncrossed. This 'openness' indicates a receptive demeanour where someone is interested in communicating and ready to listen.

Mirroring

When engaged in a deep conversation or in a conversation with someone you admire, your body will move in a way which mirrors the other person's movement. This is also referred to as a postural echo. It is a form of non-verbal communication where the gestures and the way a person is sitting or standing are copied, either consciously or subconsciously. This can create a feeling of empathy with the other person.

Proxemics or personal space

We all walk around in our own invisible 'bubble' of personal space, and we start to feel anxious or uncomfortable when someone gets too close to that bubble or penetrates it completely by touching us. Hall (1977) explored the concept of personal space and concluded that there are four zones of personal space (see Figure 1.2).

*The **intimate zone*** is reserved for those we like well and with whom we are comfortable, such as family members and lovers.

*The **personal zone*** is for those we know quite well but remain comfortable with, such as friends and close colleagues.

*The **social-consultative zone*** is for those we know reasonably well, such as more distant work colleagues or the friend of a friend.

*The **public zone*** is for everyone else, who you might know or not. You have some control over this, but it is limited. You choose when and where you go and so essentially choose what type of person is likely to be in the public area around you.

The Covid-19 pandemic has impacted our awareness of personal space and our proximity to others. With the onset of social distancing, the awareness of ourselves in relation to proximity has become more conscious and purposeful. In Activity 1.4, we will consider how personal space might feel to a patient and how, as nursing associate, you would prepare a patient for you to enter their personal space.

Activity 1.4 Reflection

Imagine yourself in a cubicle of a busy Accident and Emergency (A&E) department, waiting to be seen by a doctor. The curtains of your cubicle are closed. Now imagine yourself lying down on your back on a standard A&E trolley, with your eyes closed.

You listen and hear the general hustle and bustle of the department with some familiar and unfamiliar sounds and voices. Are you feeling relaxed at this point? Probably not.

Still with your eyes closed, you hear a curtain swish open, but you are not sure whether this is the curtain to your cubicle or one close by. Your anxiety levels are likely increasing at this point as you wait to hear what comes next. You wait and nothing happens, and slowly your anxiety levels drop a bit as you realise it must have been the

(Continued)

(Continued)

curtain to another cubicle. At that moment, someone coughs loudly near your ear, puts their hand under your shirt, from the top, and then places something cold on your chest.

What do you think your anxiety levels would be now?

How do you think you would feel?

Now think about you as the nursing associate caring for the patient we have described above. What steps would you take reduce their anxiety?

An outline answer is provided at the end of the chapter.

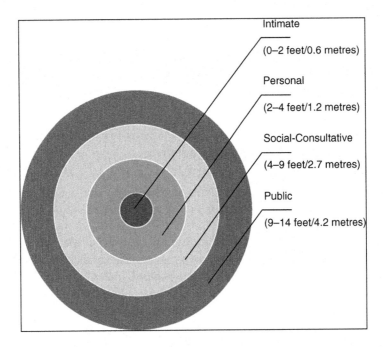

Figure 1.2   Personal space zones for middle-class North Americans of northern European heritage. Adapted from Hall (1977).

How personal space is defined and delineated varies between individuals and indeed countries. Figure 1.2 focuses on a limited group, and more recent research has attempted greater comparison. For example, Sorokowska et al. (2017) found that people from South America, in general, require less personal space than people from Asia. In addition, personal space can be variable depending on experiences and expectations. Someone who lives in a city is more likely to have a smaller overall zone than someone who lives in a more rural environment, due to the differences in human capacity between those two environments.

There are obvious exceptions to the zone 'rules', such as when we get our hair cut or step onto a busy train carriage or into a lift. In Activity 1.4, you were able to reflect on the vulnerability of patients in A&E and have hopefully come to realise that in healthcare, these exceptions become particularly important. We can be relative strangers to our patients, but we often inhabit the intimate zone. This requires real trust on behalf of the patient for them to allow us so close. This trust should be respected and never taken for granted. Our title and our appearance in a uniform gives us a unique rank of professional responsibility that permits zone mobility without question. Uniforms themselves convey a powerful dynamic and give health professionals more authority, which influences people to conform to our instructions; we must be aware of this power and use it appropriately.

Touch and the study of touch (haptics)

Touch is established as a basic human need; from the moment we are born and until death, we need to touch others and be touched. Touch is critical to our psychological, physical, emotional and social wellbeing. This is best described and most acutely seen with the initial skin to skin contact a mother and her newborn baby have. Skin to skin contact between the mother and baby:

- calms and relaxes both mother and baby;
- comforts the baby after the trauma of birth and the initial crying;
- regulates the baby's heart rate and breathing, helping them to better adapt to life outside the womb;
- stimulates digestion and an interest in feeding;
- regulates temperature;
- enables colonisation of the baby's skin with the mother's friendly bacteria, which provide protection against infection;
- stimulates the release of hormones to support breastfeeding and mothering;
- improves oxygen saturation;
- reduces cortisol (stress) levels, particularly following painful procedures;
- stimulates oxytocin, 'the love hormone' that assists with bonding (a hug lasting more than 20 seconds stimulates oxytocin);
- stimulates the natural antidepressant, serotonin;
- stimulates the pleasure chemical, dopamine.

(UNICEF, 2019)

Touch in communication is essential in forming connections and can be categorised into five types:

1. functional/professional;
2. social/polite;
3. friendship/warmth;
4. love/intimacy;
5. sexual/arousal.

(Johnson, 1988)

Some people really don't like the idea of being touched, and we, of course, need to respect those wishes, but we have to recognise that touch is fundamental, even if that touch is in the form of petting an animal. We derive pleasure from contact and an absence of contact can lead to touch starvation (Caplan, 2014). Touch starvation can be identified through a feeling of intense loneliness, depression, anxiety, stress and a difficulty sleeping.

As nursing associates, you can be defined as 'professional touchers'; that is to say, you are expected to use touch as part of your work. We can also employ therapeutic touch (also called non-contact therapeutic touch) as part of the art of nursing, where hands can be used as a form of complementary or alternative medicine. It works on the premise that a practitioner passes their hands over, or gently touches, a patient, so that their combined physical energy can cause relief (Meehan, 2001).

Appearance and smell

Appearance in relation to how we express ourselves in what we choose to wear or how we choose to present ourselves sends social messages (Eunson, 2015). Appearance and what we adorn or decorate ourselves with can communicate and carry messages about our place in society, our religion and culture, our wealth, our interest and hobbies, our occupation and much more.

Much of what we do in terms of judging people on their appearance/smell alone is superficial and subjective, coming from our own experiences and biases.

A bias is a form of prejudice for or against something, someone or a particular group, often in comparison to another group or individual. This bias may have a positive or negative outcome depending on what the bias means for you. There are two types of bias:

1.   conscious bias (also known as *explicit*/clear and obvious bias);
2.   unconscious bias (also known as *implicit*/indirect or unintentional bias).

When we hear words like 'prejudice' in relation to biases, there is an easy assumption that this is specific to race and ethnicity, but biases exist towards any range of identifiable criteria, such as age, gender, disability, sexual orientation, religion, weight or hair colour. There is no end to the characteristics that could be subject to a bias.

Unconscious or implicit biases are learned stereotypes that are automatic, unintentional, often deeply set and can easily influence our behaviour. They are triggers without thought and are reactive elements of our personality (Oberai and Anand, 2018). Within healthcare, the unconscious bias can be very damaging and lead to discrimination. Reflecting on our biases and challenging them is essential for delivering non-judgemental and non-discriminatory care. In Chapter 6, we will discuss bias and discrimination in more detail.

Written

Written communication is a method of getting a message across in writing. This can be through letters, whether handwritten or typed, pamphlets, booklets or electronic means, via websites with words, emails or text messages. It is a less flexible, formal means of communication.

We explore professional communication further in Chapter 2.

Visual

Visual communication involves the use of symbols and images to get a message across. It is the most universal means of communication and is an easily shared and relied upon method. It uses signs, graphics, films, photographs and many other methods. A good example is the use of toilet door signage as a means of directing people.

We explore visual communication further in Chapter 7.

The theory of communication

Understanding the theory of communication and the underlying barriers and observations makes you a more able communicator. It allows you to explore and reflect on your own communication style, to consider what makes good or bad communication possible.

The very first recorded communication theory was formulated by the Greek philosopher Aristotle, who, unencumbered by technology, and addressing a population who were mostly illiterate, had a simple model. It consisted of just three elements: a speaker, a message and a listener or audience. In 1948, the political scientist Harold Laswell expanded on this to include a 'medium' or mode of delivery of the message.

Universally, the study of communication examines the development and structure of language. To begin with, the language studied was the mathematical language used in computer programming.

Shannon and Weaver's model

Shannon and Weaver's model (1948) was initially developed to explore communication in the context of the telecommunications industry. The 'sender' and 'receiver' in this instance refers to hardware and not individuals. There are, however, clear parallels for this model to be applied to direct human communication.

Shannon and Weaver's model is an example of a linear or straight-lined model. You can see from Figure 1.3 that there is a clear direction from the sender to the receiver, and, importantly in this model, there is a mechanism for feedback from the receiver to the sender. This process is, however, rigid and does not support a more fluid, dynamic interaction that is needed in an exchange of views.

What this model does do well is in acknowledging 'noise' as a barrier to communication. A busy hospital ward, or waiting room, with its unfamiliar buzzers, announcements and ringing telephones, will influence how a message will be received.

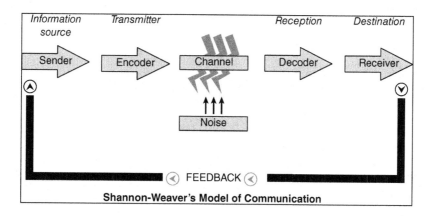

Figure 1.3 Shannon and Weaver's model of communication.

Considering the environment where communication takes place will increase the potential success of a communication.

As the nursing associate wanting to discuss a topic with a patient, you are the sender or the information source. How you decide to transmit the information then makes you the encoder. This information is channelled between you and the patient as the receiver. For the patient to receive the message as you intended to share it, they must be able to decode the information accurately without any distortion or interference.

Berlo's model

In 1960, Berlo further developed Shannon and Weaver's mathematical communication theory. Berlo's SMCR model of communication work was the first of its kind intended to look at the 'ingredients' of effective communication, which included human characteristics. Using the information theory approach, Berlo broke down the stages of a standard communication process. Specifically, he identified that there must be a source (S) or sender of the communication, and that there must be a message (M) to send. He then considered the way or channel (C) chosen by the sender by which to give the message. Finally, he recognised the role of the receiver (R) in getting that message.

The SMCR model of communication can therefore be broken down as another linear model (see Figure 1.4).

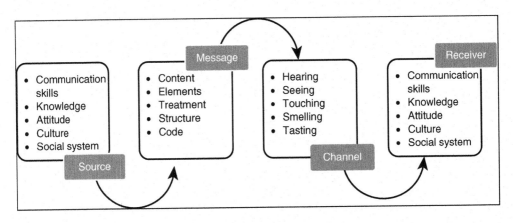

Figure 1.4   Adapted from the Berlo model (1960).

Source

Communication skills refers to the ability and competence of the sender to express the message. It takes into account their ability to read, write and speak.

Knowledge recognises that the source or sender must understand what the message is going to be and have a sound grasp of the subject or topic.

Attitude explores the opinion the source has about themselves, the subject and those they are communicating to. For example, if the source needed to send a message about a topic they disagreed with, this would influence how and what they chose to communicate.

Culture includes consideration of the values, beliefs, religion and experiences a person has had. As an example, a person raised following the faith of Jehovah Witnesses would not permit the use of blood products as treatment for themselves, but they do recognise that blood products can be used for individuals who hold a different set of beliefs.

Message

Content refers to the entire message from start to finish, from the moment the communication starts to the final word uttered, heard or read.

The model considers the various techniques in communication, such as the language used, eye contact, the use of touch and gestures.

Treatment is the way in which the message is conveyed. An example here is when using a pamphlet written in English with someone who can only speak Urdu. This would be an ineffective means of communication. Tailoring the message to the needs of the receiver is a much more effective way to communicate.

Structure refers to the way in which the message has been structured. It explores whether the information is logically presented and therefore easily understood.

Code looks at what form the message is sent through. It could be through body language, speech, sign language, gestures, music, dance or in writing, to name a few.

Channel

The channel is the way the message is sent and how the message will be received using one or more of the five senses, focusing on the sensory system of the receiver. It may therefore involve sight, sound, smell, taste or touch.

Receiver

In Berlo's model, the receiver is subject to the same factors that the source has that affect and influence the sending of the message.

This linear approach assumes that the source or sender and the receiver have similar attitudes, understanding and experiences. In a healthcare context, this is rarely the case, when we, as the experienced healthcare professional, are communicating our specialist knowledge to a patient with limited medical knowledge.

This difference in experience can lead to misunderstandings and misinterpretation of the message. Berlo's model does not consider any barriers to communication and does not allow for feedback to check understanding. It also fails to appreciate any outside influences on communication due to the environment, such as noise in the background.

Schramm's model

Wilbur Schramm's model (1954) introduced the circular design in communication theory, recognising the importance of how both the sender and the receiver *interpret* the message, rather than solely focusing on the sender's meaning of the message. He explored the concept that communication is circular and not a linear mechanism only going in one direction; it is a two-way process whereby the sender and the receiver are delivering a message and giving feedback as a simultaneous active process.

Another key development with the Schramm model (see Figure 1.5) is the acknowledgement that there needs to be an overlap between the sender and the receiver's field of experience. Without even the smallest overlap in experiences or a degree of a meeting of minds, communication is very difficult, if not impossible. Applying the field of experience means that this model is best used by two individuals in a dialogue together and cannot be applied to large groups.

A criticism of this model is that it implies an equality in the communication. Very often, communication in healthcare settings with patients is unbalanced. The presence of a person in uniform can be intimidating and the medical terminology is hard for some people to interpret. This is particularly the case if we factor in communication resources, power, and time given to communicate the imbalance (Mcquail and Windhall, 2015, p. 20).

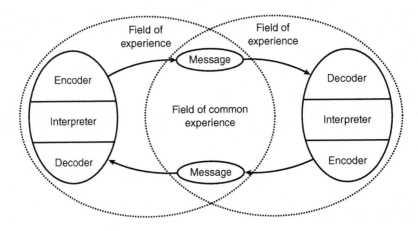

Figure 1.5 Schramm's model.

Riley and Riley's mass communication model

It is important to recognise that, as nursing associates, your communication is not going to be restricted to one-to-one or small group interactions. There will be a need to communicate with larger groups too. Riley and Riley's model (1959) (see Figure 1.6) of mass communication is a transactional model where the communicator (C) is part of a larger social system, such as a body of nurses and nursing associates.

The Riley and Riley model shows that the communicator sends information and messages according to the needs and expectations of a group of people receiving (R) the information. The group of people have formed in a similar social structure, such as a group of patients.

There is a clear two-way basis of communication where both (C) and (R) are parts of and represent a large social system. We can see that both groups are part of an overall social system; both the communicator and receiver are dependent on the interaction

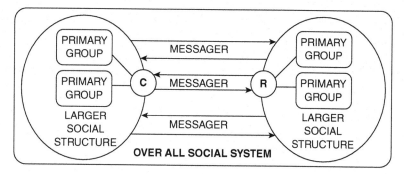

Figure 1.6   Riley and Riley (1959).

and the feedback. This model helps to create a better understanding between the groups and helps to resolve disputes.

Key stages in any communication from any model

Whether using a circular (transactional) or linear model, there remain some agreement that all communications involve three key steps. An understanding of each step and what goes into it will enable you to communicate more effectively with patients, carers and the multidisciplinary team (MDT).

These steps are:

Encoding

When getting a message ready to send, we need to think about how we are going to do this so that we get our message across clearly and effectively. We think about the words we are going to use or the tools we are going to employ. We organise our thoughts and consider how the message will be received.

Decoding

Following the receipt of a message, we need to make sense of it and draw some meaning from the message.

Interpreting

Once you have found the meaning in the message, you need to interpret what that means to you. Is it relevant? Have you understood it correctly? It is very possible that you may interpret the message one way while someone else may have a totally different interpretation of the same message, or in a different way to that which the sender or encoder intended.

Once a message has been decoded and interpreted, the receiver can become the sender and go about encoding their own message to be sent back to the original sender, and the process is repeated in the opposite direction, and so on and so forth as the cycle continues! You will go through these stages of communication countless times a day in your role as nursing associate, often without even thinking about it.

Chapter summary

In this chapter, you have been introduced to the subject of communication, looking at how and why we communicate and how models of communication have evolved to try and address the complexity of interpersonal communication. We have explored communication from a basic level of subconscious activity to consciously planned and prepared communications which alter in complexity.

As nursing associates, it is essential to get a grasp of these aspects of communication and the impact they have on our day-to-day living, as well as the impact they have on those with whom we communicate, whether they be a child who only has a vocabulary of a few words, an elderly person with cognitive impairments or the members of our healthcare teams. It is key to our success and integral to good care delivery.

Activities: Brief outline answers

Activity 1.1 Critical thinking (page 3)

What would happen? I would expect that the birds would immediately fly away and scatter in response to the sound.

Why? A loud noise or unexpected event associated with a loud noise would stimulate a fight and flight response in the pigeons, who would interpret the situation as a dangerous one in which they need to escape. It is a method of self-preservation.

Similarly, the family would also react. They would be startled by the unexpected and loud noise and would immediately investigate the situation, seeking the source of the noise to explore whether they need to flee any danger too, not unlike our feathered friends.

Activity 1.2 Reflection (page 4)

Verbal examples: face-to-face talking (either with an individual or a group), over the telephone, video recording, voice recording.

Non-verbal examples: facial expressions, body language, posture, eye contact, touch.

Written examples: emails, letters, text messages, posters, PowerPoint presentations, white boards, information booklets, handwriting.

Visual examples: photographs, video recording, charts, graphs, drawing, art, sketches, models, dioramas.

Activity 1.3 Work-based learning (page 5)

IM	Intra muscular	EEG	Electroencephalogram	Stat	Straight away
TPR	Temperature, pulse and respiration	ECG	Electrocardiogram	#	Fracture
BNO	Bowels not open	QDS	Four times a day	CXR	Chest x-ray
NBM	Nil by mouth	PRN	As needed	DNAR	Do not attempt resuscitation

Figure 1.7   Common medical abbreviations: answers.

Activity 1.4 Reflection (page 9)

'What do you think your anxiety levels would be now?' It is likely you thought your anxiety levels would be very high at this point.

'How do you think you would feel?' You may also have said that you were feeling vulnerable and scared too.

'Now think about you as the nursing associate caring for the patient we have described above. What steps would you take reduce their anxiety?' It is important to introduce yourself to the patient in the first instance and then manage the expectations of the patient. Where a patient has impaired senses, as with the scenario you were asked to imagine, communication of your actions is vital to reduce anxiety.

When the curtain was pulled back, the practitioner entering the cubicle was entering the social-consultative zone and they should have introduced themselves to the patient. As the practitioner moved closer to the patient, they entered the personal zone. This is where a dialogue or description of what is going to happen next should have taken place, and consent should have been established prior to entering the intimate zone and touching the patient. The practitioner should then explain their actions, saying something like: 'I am going to place my hand under the top of your shirt and listen to your chest. The equipment I will use to do this will be a little cold.'

Then the role of the practitioner is to close the interaction and offer a timeframe and an explanation of the next steps in their care, while giving the patient an opportunity to ask questions.

Knowledge review

Now that you have worked through the chapter, how would you rate your knowledge of the following topics?

	Good	Adequate	Poor
1. the definition of communication			
2. different types of communication			

	Good	Adequate	Poor
3. the development of communication theory			
4. models of communication			
5. how we communicate			

If you are unsure of some aspects, what are you going to do next?

Further reading and useful websites

For more information on the communication theories discussed in this chapter, and to explore other theories, go to:
www.communicationtheory.org/

An excellent resource from the Royal College of Nursing on non-verbal communication:
https://rcni.com/hosted-content/rcn/first-steps/non-verbal-communication

Find out more about transforming care for babies, their mothers and their families:
www.unicef.org.uk/babyfriendly/about/standards/

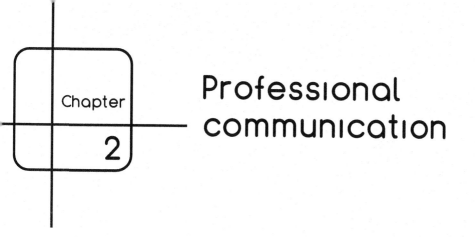

Chapter 2

Professional communication

NMC FUTURE NURSE STANDARDS OF PROFICIENCY FOR NURSING ASSOCIATES

This chapter will address the following platforms and proficiencies:

Platform 1: Being an accountable professional

At the point of registration, the nursing associate will be able to:

1.9   communicate effectively using a range of skills and strategies with colleagues and people at all stages of life and with a range of mental, physical, cognitive and behavioural health challenges.

1.10   demonstrate the skills and abilities required to develop, manage and maintain appropriate relationships with people, their families, carers and colleagues.

1.14   demonstrate the ability to keep complete, clear, accurate and timely records.

Platform 3: Provide and monitor care

At the point of registration, the nursing associate will be able to:

3.11   demonstrate the ability to recognise when a person's condition has improved or deteriorated by undertaking health monitoring. Interpret, promptly respond, share findings, and escalate as needed.

3.18   demonstrate the ability to monitor the effectiveness of care in partnership with people, families and carers. Document progress and report outcomes.

Platform 4: Working in teams

At the point of registration, the nursing associate will be able to:

4.4   demonstrate the ability to effectively and responsibly access, input and apply information and data using a range of methods including digital technologies, and share appropriately within interdisciplinary teams.

(Continued)

(Continued)

4.8   contribute to team reflection activities, to promote improvements in practice and services.

Annexe A: Communication and relationship management skills

At the point of registration, the nursing associate will be able to safely demonstrate the following skills:

4.   Communication skills for working in professional teams:

Demonstrate effective skills when working in teams through:

4.1   active listening when receiving feedback and when dealing with team members' concerns and anxieties.
4.2   timely and appropriate escalation.
4.3   being a calm presence when exposed to situations involving conflict.
4.4   being assertive when required.
4.5   using de-escalation strategies and techniques when dealing with conflict.

5.   Demonstrate effective supervision skills by providing:

5.1   clear instructions and explanations when supervising others.
5.2   clear instructions and checking understanding when delegating care responsibilities to others.
5.3   clear constructive feedback in relation to care delivered by others.
5.4   encouragement to colleagues that helps them to reflect on their practice.

Chapter aims

By the end of this chapter, you will be able to:

- discuss the ways in which we share information.
- explore the correct use of the telephone and verbal, in-person, handovers.
- understand the importance of note keeping.
- understand the dangers of social media.
- gain some insight into confidentiality.

Introduction

In the previous chapter, we looked at the ways in which we communicate and some of the theories we can use in communicating. Now we are moving on to professional communication and its significance in the role of the nursing associate. In this chapter, the variety of ways in which information is shared, delivered or interpreted will be explored. This will include learning to share information by email and text message, using technological advancements in communication, and the possible dangers of social media. This chapter will also include case studies to illustrate how giving information, using correct telephone etiquette, verbal handovers and maintaining confidentiality can be applied in practice. The four themes of *The Code* (NMC, 2018a) will also be discussed because nursing associates will be required to uphold them in order to register and practise in the UK.

Definition

So, you want to be a professional? Let's look at what this means. Being a professional means that you are a member of a group of people who perform or engage in skilled and learned activities which require a specialist knowledge. For nursing associates, there is an additional element to being a professional, and that is being registered with the professional regulatory and statuary body, which in our case is the NMC; specifically, we are bound to promote professionalism and trust (NMC, 2018a), and when we register with the NMC, we agree to conform to the technical and ethical standards of the profession.

As you have already seen at the start of this chapter, the NMC puts a significant emphasis on registrants being able to practise effectively (NMC, 2018a) and communicate not only with patients, clients and their significant others, but as part of a local team of colleagues from a variety of specialisms and professional backgrounds, as well as to a wider healthcare community, including volunteers, charities and inter-agency collaborations, who all require professional communication.

Communicating professionally in a healthcare setting requires an understanding of the variety of roles and responsibilities of the multidisciplinary team (MDT). It also means building appropriate relationships to allow for the exchange of knowledge and skills. This will enable the effective delivery of care to our service user/patient group (Kenaszchuk et al., 2010).

As nursing associates, you will form a unique and recently explored route in communication within the professional team and between patients and clients. The newness of the nursing associate role can be a challenge when integrating into established teams and long-established healthcare professional roles. From the very beginning of its development, it was thought that the nursing associate role would be the essential bridge between registered nurses and doctors and those being cared for, not only in terms of the more direct nature of your caring role with patients and clients, but essentially in terms of communication.

Nursing associates work cooperatively with the registered nurses and other healthcare professionals in providing and monitoring care delivery. During a four-day inpatient stay in hospital, it is estimated that the patient will have contact with at least 50 different employees, from catering and housekeeping staff to nurses, technicians and doctors (O'Daniel and Rosenstein, 2008). As the professional healthcare worker with the biggest potential for actual hands-on working with patients and clients, the nursing associate role is to coordinate and facilitate contacts with your patient and service user group. This should be done in a way which ensures safety, dignity, respect, compassion and, of course, care.

Sharing information in a professional way

Recognising someone as a professional is to acknowledge their conduct, experience, quality and study of their topic, which in this situation is healthcare. As nursing associates, you are a professional in your own right and are able to make a significant contribution to effective clinical practices.

Communicating as a team of professionals is essential. When healthcare professionals fail to communicate effectively, it has a direct effect on the safety of patient care. There are many ways in which this can happen. A lack of critical information or the misinterpretation or misunderstanding of information, for example, from unclear telephone orders or poor handwriting and grammar, can mean critical information is lost or overlooked. As registrants with the NMC (2018a), we are bound to preserve safety, so it is essential that we get our communication right.

Spelling and grammar

There is an old saying that you can't read a doctor's writing. Thankfully, now with the engagement of technology and typing, messages are more clearly communicated and miscommunications are limited. However, there are still situations where handwriting is commonly used. Handwriting must be legible, words must be spelled correctly, and all writing must contain accurate grammar and punctuation. If you are unsure what has been written, you must check with the person who wrote it before any action is taken or any medication is given. As you can appreciate, if you give the wrong drug because you have misread it and did not check, there would be severe consequences.

Verbal orders via the telephone

Verbal orders are when a prescriber gives an oral/verbal instruction, usually via the telephone to a nurse to record or amend a prescription and then administer it. Verbal orders are associated with a high number of medication errors and should only be used in exceptional circumstances. As an example, if you confuse Doxepin (oral tricyclic anti-depressive, standard dose of 75 milligrams (mg)) and Digoxin (a potent drug which treats atrial fibrillation and heart failure, where the standard daily dose is 125 micrograms (mcg)), the consequences would be grave.

Verbal orders are permitted for use only when any delay in administering a medication would compromise patient care (Royal Pharmaceutical Society, 2019). A study in a large psychiatric hospital asked 50 nurses if they would take a verbal order from a doctor over the telephone; 26% said they would not take the verbal order. On questioning, only 12% of the 50 nurses that where asked were aware of the current guidance. A further 12% stated that they lacked confidence in taking a verbal order or were unsure of the exact procedure, while 62% were unable to correctly describe how to take a verbal order (Hall et al., 2014).

It is important to follow your employer's policy for verbal orders, which will be found on either hard copy in the place of work or via the local intranet. Where verbal orders are permitted, the prescriber ordering the change is responsible for writing the new prescription or amending the details of the prescription as soon as possible, ideally within 24 hours. If this is not possible, the prescriber is responsible for ensuring that the patient's records are updated electronically (Royal Pharmaceutical Society, 2019).

As nursing associates, and so as a NMC registrant, you could be in the position of taking a verbal order. It is therefore essential that you get that order checked with another registrant before any medication is administered. If in any doubt, check again. Activity 2.1 asks you to practise your pronunciation skills and challenges your ability to listen to the names of different drugs that are in common use.

Activity 2.1   Communication: listening and pronunciation

This activity is best done with a colleague; take turns to read out loud the following pairs of drug names and write down what you hear:

1. Doxepin (Dox – ee – pin)

    Digoxin (Dij – ox – in)

2. Clobazam (Clo – baz – am)

    Clonazepam (Clon – as – a – pam)

    Both drugs are used for the treatment of epilepsy, but they both have very different doses.

3. Sulfadiazine (Sul – fa – die – a – zeen)

    Sulfasalazine (Sul – fa – sall – a – zeen)

    Sulfadiazine is indicated for the prevention of rheumatic fever, whereas Sulfasalazine is used in the treatment of:

*   mild to moderate and severe ulcerative colitis and maintenance of remission active Crohn's disease;
*   rheumatoid arthritis.

4. Mercaptamine (Mer – cap – ta – mean)

    Mercaptopurine (Mer – cap – toe – purr – in)

    Mercaptamine is used for the treatment of proven nephropathic cystinosis (a rare disorder of the kidneys, which develops in young children). Mercaptopurine is used for the treatment of leukaemia.

    Can you think of any other drug names which may cause confusion? Reflect on your experience of listening and reading the drug names out loud. More information on drug safety and drug name confusion can be found on the gov.uk website at the end of the chapter.

As this is a verbal activity, there is no suggested model answer.

Lookalike and soundalike medications are a particular problem, and healthcare is littered with long and complicated names for medications, conditions and procedures. Taking the time to practise, breaking down these words and getting them checked if you are not sure, is good practice.

It does, however, highlight the risks in taking instructions over the telephone. It would be very easy to mishear an order and put a patient at risk. The mistake may be seen as innocent, and no harm would be intended; however, as a registered nursing associate, you would remain accountable for the error regardless of the intention and may still face disciplinary action.

Verbal handovers in person

As you have seen following Activity 2.1, translating verbal orders and instructions can be difficult. Despite this, verbal handovers are a crucial communication tool and are essential to the delivery and coordination of care during the patient journey. The effectiveness of verbal handovers – how they are done, what should be included in them and what skills are required to deliver a verbal handover – have been studied and discussed at length for many years. As a result, there have been many changes to the verbal handover, but none of them to date can offer the perfect solution.

The evidence from this research, however, suggests that a structured handover, which puts patients at the centre, gives rise to increased patient safety and care continuity. A further advantage is job satisfaction for the nurse or nursing associate (Ballantyne, 2017).

Essentially, a verbal handover is 'the transfer of professional responsibility and accountability for some or all aspects of care for a patient or group of patients, to another or professional group on a temporary or permanent basis' (National Patient Safety Agency et al., 2004). There is a tendency to think about handover only happening at the shift change time, but we hand over the care and management of a patient in a variety of other situations too. Other situations where we hand over the care of a patient includes moving patients between departments when a patient needs a chest x-ray, for example, or when they are admitted to a ward from urgent care. Another common handover takes place when discharging to a nursing home or home and into the care of the community team, or directly to the patient or their carer.

We have focused here on verbal handovers because they are the typical form of handover. As with taking orders by telephone, which we saw in the previous section, there are some problems with verbal handovers. Some of the information can get lost through interference and not heard correctly.

Types of in-person verbal handovers

Office-based (closed handovers)

In a healthcare setting, when we think about a handover, we usually think of all of the nursing staff being huddled together in the ward office or any other private environment, often with a cup of tea in hand and on a mismatch of chairs. This type of handover is setting the scene for the upcoming shift. The benefits include minimising disruptions, ensuring patient confidentiality and allowing for an open discussion of sensitive topics. These topics might include test results and treatment plans which have not yet been discussed with the patient, but also might include issues such as concerns over domestic violence or mental capacity.

However, it does not include the patient, who is central to the discussion; it does not take into account the patient's feelings in real time and does not allow them to ask questions, or to be fully up to date in clinical decision making. There is also a staffing issue with an office-based handover, as it relies on there being someone available to provide care and be present on the ward for the duration of the handover. This would usually be the most junior members of the team, such as healthcare support workers and students.

In the community setting, the clinical handover may only happen on a weekly basis as part of the multidisciplinary team meeting. This leaves a crucial communication gap with those members of staff working out in the community, so it is important that there is some daily contact among the team, even if this is via the phone, and there must be agreed communication avenues for the escalation of concerns (Pearce, 2018). It is also a means of professional and emotional support for the nurses, who will be working alone for most of their working day.

Bedside handovers

Since 2015, there has been an increase in handovers taking place at the patient's bedside. These were developed in order to emphasise the involvement the patient has in their care. This is not to deny that there are benefits in an office-based handover. These bedside handovers, however, are reflective of our duty to prioritise people (NMC, 2018a), the patient's demand for information and the increased availability of information from internet sources. Patients are encouraged to inform themselves about their conditions so that they are in a better position to understand and discuss their healthcare needs.

A bedside handover is the perfect opportunity to give a full summary of the care the patient has received that day. The nurse and the patient can also discuss any clinical developments or changes and the nurse can ask the patient how they feel. Significantly, we also need to consider the language we use. If we are using technical terms, it can be very awkward if the patient does not understand the terminology; equally, we do not want to dumb down the language used and patronise the patient (Pearce, 2018). With the use of medical language, it is essential that we allow the patient and their significant others to ask questions to help clarify their understanding. Remember, there are no stupid questions; there are only stupid answers.

We do need to be mindful of our environment when we are discussing sensitive issues with a patient. There is an obvious issue of patient confidentiality with bedside handovers and the ability of the person in the next bed being able to hear the handover. The patient under discussion must be able to consent to this bedside handover. In an open ward environment, all the other patients are listening, and this could lead to sensitive topics being brushed over or not discussed at all, which would have a detrimental effect on patient care.

Outside of the issue of confidentiality, bedside handovers are problematic, due to the general hubbub of the clinical environment; phones will ring and buzzers will alarm; staff and visitors will come and go. The general daily interference takes its toll on the concentration of the staff in the handover and it may also limit the opportunities for the patients to ask any questions.

What we hand over

Regardless of the location of the handover, getting order in what is handed over is important. Using a familiar and logical format to a handover allows the listener to anticipate the type of information that will be given. It enables those giving the information to deliver a confident, structured and efficient handover without items being repeated or missed.

The tool most commonly used within the NHS is the SBAR tool.

S	**Situation** Asking: What is going on with the patient?	**An introduction** (no need to do this if you are known to the listener): • My name is (x) • I am a Nursing Associate on/in (state ward or clinical environment) **The reason for the communication** I have a query about some medication that has been prescribed (as an example) Or I would like to hand over this patient to you.
B	**Background** Asking: How did the patient come to be here?	**Brief history:** • State patient's name in full and what they may like to be called • Their age • Any other relevant past medical history • State when they were admitted (state date), from (state how they came into your care: from Accident and Emergency, or GP referral, for example), what they were admitted with (state general reason) • State what therapy/procedure/investigations they have had and when (how long ago).

A	**Assessment**
	
	Asking:
	
	What is the problem?
		Summary:
		
		• State outcome/result of therapy/procedure/investigations
		• Note any changes in their condition
		• State a summary of their observations/urine output/bowels (open/ or not)/pain status/diet and hydration/level of alertness (if being measured)
		
		   o can use the A–E assessment tool for this*
		   o AVPU**
		   o NEWS (2)***
		
		• State any social issues (if relevant)
		• Make a general summary of their care at this current time.
		
		(For example, if their temperature has gone up and they look flushed and hot, you could comment that you think they might have an infection.)

R	**Recommendations** Asking: What is going to happen next for this patient?	**Plan:** • State what interventions are needed (if any) (such as take blood/ repeat the chest x-ray/call the doctor) • Include any recommendations from wider multidisciplinary team (such as physiotherapy twice a week/referral to occupational therapy) • State date/time for next review of the patient.
Encourage questions and get listener to repeat key information to ensure that it is understood.		

Figure 2.1 Work-based learning.

The SBAR tool (see Figure 2.1) originated from the US Navy and was adapted for use in healthcare by Dr M. Leonard and colleagues from Kaiser Permanente, Colorado, USA.

Additional information from SBAR

1. A to E assessment consists of a summary of the following:

    A – Airway

    B – Breathing

    C – Circulation

    D – Disability

    E – Exposure

2. AVPU (see Figure 2.1) to the assessment of states of consciousness:

    A – Alert

    V – Verbal

    P – Pain

    U – Unresponsive

3. NEWS (see Figure 2.1) is the National Early Warning Score. NEWS2 is for use in acute care settings or ambulance settings.

The NEWS score is calculated from information from the patient's respiratory rate, oxygen saturations, whether they are on oxygen, their temperature, the systolic blood pressure, heart rate and the level of consciousness.

In Activity 2.2, you are being asked to look at some general information that would be given as part of an SBAR handover.

Activity 2.2   Case study

How would you hand over this patient using the SBAR tool (you might want to think about the order of the information in the case study to make the handover more logical)?

A patient had a total abdominal **hysterectomy** and **bilateral salpingo oophorectomy**. Her name is Mrs Choudhary; she had the operation one week ago, and she likes to be called Swarda. Her ECG was fine, but she has a raised temperature. She is 57 years old and has a Robinson drain in on the right side. Urine output dropped. Her pain is relieved with patient-controlled analgesia and she has not had her bowels open. She is nil by mouth and has a nasogastric tube (plugged) and an IV with fluid (dextrose and saline). Wound draining a lot. All started with abdominal pain for two weeks.

An outline answer is provided at the end of the chapter.

Keeping notes and medical records

Thinking about the previous section and the case study specifically in Activity 2.2, and making reference to the jargon buster activity in Chapter 1, it is not hard to see why medicine has developed its own form of code or shorthand. Writing everything out in full without the agreed abbreviations would be very time consuming, not only to write but also to read. If you found yourself in an emergency and you needed a summary of the patient quickly, the medical shorthand in the notes helps you navigate the situation quickly. Now try Activity 2.3.

Activity 2.3   Communication

Try to decode these two patient record notes:

1. 57 o+, 1/7 post TAH BSO, PCA insitu, i/c Robinson   (R)

    wound +++ >temp ECG NAD, <PU, IV (Dex/Sal), NBM, NGT, BNO, TEDs

2. 35 O->, 6/7 post RTC # Bil Tib/Fib, O$_2$ 50% resp 25, 2° turns, PMH asthma, nebs QDS

An outline answer is provided at the end of the chapter.

As you have seen from Activity 2.3, there is a benefit to using medical shorthand. It must not be offensive and must be easily translatable, for a court of law or for an application for access to medical records request (Access to the Medical Act (1990)). If you keep pocket notes to remind you of the tasks you have to complete, these must not have any identifiable details on them which would be in breach of the General Data Protection Regulations (GDPR) (HMSO, 2018). These handwritten pocket notes must be transcribed into the relevant medical notes within 24 hours and securely destroyed.

As a nursing associate, you will be responsible for writing in the nursing notes; essentially, you must provide a factual, consistent, accurate and clear account of the care provided and the condition of the patient. Using a standardised format will help with consistency and the quality of the record and should include assessments, plans and the implementation of the plan and the evaluation of care. As much as these aspects are situation and patient specific, there are some general rules to follow:

- It sounds simple, but make sure that you are writing in the correct notes. Check the patient's person data. Question, is this the right name? Is this the right date of birth? Is this their correct address? It is rare, but it does happen that you have two patients in at the same time with the same name.
- Notes must be promptly recorded. However, if you do have to add something after the fact, you need to state that it is a 'retrospective account'.
- What you add to records must not be erased or deleted without notice. Never scribble out notes or cover up. If you write something in error, you must state

'written in error', including the date, time, your signature and your position of nursing associate.

- Similarly with alterations, you must state 'altered record' followed by the date, time, signature and position.
- Limit the jargon and abbreviations in nursing notes. No meaningless phrases, irrelevant information, no speculation or offensive comments.

   o   Avoid phrases such as 'appeared well', 'all care given', 'care as per care plan', 'slept well'.

- The notes must be accurately dated and timed using the 24-hour clock (for example, 14:00 instead of 2 p.m.) and signed with your signature alongside a printed version of your name and your role, as the record keeper.
- If the record is handwritten, it must be readable when photocopied. Use dark ink (ideally black) and keep notes out of direct sunlight.
- If a problem is identified, you must state what you did about it.
- You must provide clear evidence of the care delivered.

Just because something has not been written down does not mean that it did not happen. Often, what you fail to write is as telling as what you do write. For example, if you made a drug error and did not record it anywhere, it does not mean that the drug error did not happen. It just means that you kept it a secret and were dishonest. Own your mistakes wherever possible, so that you and others can learn from them and make sure that they don't happen again.

The use of social media

When done right, the use of social media sites, in whatever form, can be a fantastic way of keeping in touch with old friends, new trends and relevant nursing and professional issues. It has the potential to be a positive, rewarding and informative experience.

However, with the increasing number of NMC registrants being subject to charges at fitness to practise panels for the inappropriate use of social media, it is clear that of the estimated 355,000 registered nurses and midwives using Facebook (Osborne, 2012), some of us are getting it really quite wrong. In Activity 2.4, you are asked to think about professional conduct and boundaries when it comes to using social media sites.

Activity 2.4   Case study: social media

You are working in the community and have been visiting a 31-year-old man. He is paraplegic after a sporting injury. He lives with his parents, and you have provided care with his bowel and catheter care on a weekly basis for the last nine months. After your last visit, you notice that he has sent you a friend request via one of your social media platforms. You are due to visit him again in two days' time. What do you think is the best response to his friend request?

An outline answer is provided at the end of the chapter.

As we have seen in Activity 2.4, social media is difficult to control and predict. Seven staff from the Great Western Hospital in Swindon were suspended in 2009 after posting pictures of themselves playing a viral game called 'the lying down game', which involved being photographed lying face down in unusual places. The doctors and nurses from the A&E department photographed each other in a variety of places, which included resuscitation trolleys, ward floors and on the Wiltshire air ambulance helipad. These pictures were then posted on a social media site where they were seen by the hospital management (Press Association, 2009).

The NMC (2010), in their guidance on the responsible use of social media, stated that:

Nurses, midwives and nursing associates may put their registration at risk, and students may jeopardise their ability to join our register, if they act in any way that is unprofessional or unlawful on social media, including (but not limited to):

- sharing confidential information inappropriately;
- posting pictures of patients and people receiving care without their consent;
- posting inappropriate comments about patients;
- bullying, intimidating or exploiting people;
- building or pursuing relationships with patients or service users;
- stealing personal information or using someone else's identity;
- encouraging violence or self-harm;
- inciting hatred or discrimination.

As human beings, we are not perfect, and our petty annoyances often need to be aired and shared. But you must be cautious when using the remoteness of a computer or social media site to share any grievances, even if they are shared as a private message. Inappropriate private behaviour is still inappropriate behaviour and will be treated as such if it breaches the NMC ruling.

Being in a trusted position as a nursing associate, you are free to access personal and private details of the patients and clients you work with. Any inappropriate disclosure of those details, or the use of those details for your personal use, is against the law. General Data Protection Regulation (GDPR) (2018 amended 2019) clearly states how personal information can be shared, and it is important that you follow the strict data protection principles.

You must make sure of the following:

- The information must be used fairly, lawfully and transparently.
- Sharing of information must be for a specified or explicit purpose.
- Personal data should be used in a way that is adequate, relevant and limited to only what is necessary.
- The information must be accurate and, where necessary, kept up to date.
- Any information shared should be kept for no longer than is necessary.
- Information should be handled in a way that ensures appropriate security, including protection against unlawful or unauthorised processing, access, loss, destruction or damage.

There is stronger legal protection for more sensitive information, such as information relevant to ethnicity, race, health, sex or sexual orientation and any political or religious beliefs.

In addition to GDPR, under Article 8 of the European Convention of Human Rights (1998), we have a right to privacy, and as healthcare professionals, you have an obligation not to abuse your power when it comes to accessing information. Activity 2.5 explores a nurse's or nursing associate's inappropriate use of a patient's personal information.

Activity 2.5   Critical thinking

A registered adult nurse was struck off the NMC register in August 2018, while working in a hospital in Lancashire. The nurse accessed a patient's personal details and used them to follow that patient on more than one social media forum. The nurse made contact with the patient to invite them to their house and then on holiday. The nurse had previously touched the patient inappropriately while in their care and at the NMC hearing, the registrant admitted that their actions were sexually motivated.

Think about how you would feel if you were the patient. What impact does the nurse's actions have on the hospital they worked in?

An outline answer is provided at the end of the chapter.

Protect yourself

As explored in Activity 2.5, it is important to maintain professional boundaries when using social media. It is also essential that you are aware of how you share your information on social media too, so you can protect yourself.

As nursing associates, some of your personal information is freely available to the public or whoever wants to find us. A quick, free search using my first name and surname on the NMC website will give the reader my middle name (it is Louise, by the way), my general location, when I joined the register and when I qualified as a teacher of nurses.

When you think about our accessibility, we can also consider our vulnerability too. If you look down your lists of friends on any particular social media platform, how many of them would you consider to be actual friends, who you could trust with your information and your pictures? Are you certain that of those friends, their friends are just as reliable?

It is easy for posted content to get out of your control very quickly, and before you may know it, you are the next viral sensation. It is important that you consider whom you associate with and what you may endorse by association. Even historical posts can be resurrected and used out of context to cast a shadow over your professionalism.

We just need to think of the case of Rebecca Leighton, who was a nurse falsely accused of poisoning some patients while employed at Stepping Hill Hospital in 2011. During the investigation, some of the UK newspapers found photographs of Miss Leighton on a social media site and used the pictures out of context in newspaper articles. The pictures chosen painted an image of her which was one of recklessness, aggression and someone who was flirty. One image in particular would appear to have been taken at a fancy-dress party, where she was a cowboy. The toy gun was prominent in the picture, which leads the reader to associate her with a weapon, next to photographs of some of the victims. These images lead to her being dubbed 'The Angel of Death', and she was reported as being so scared for her life that she could not go out. Although innocent, she had a trial by media, assisted by her own pictures from a social media site. The actual killer was Victorino Chua, who was sentenced to life in prison in 2015.

In Activity 2.6, we look into simple steps you can take to protect yourself on social media platforms.

Activity 2.6   Critical thinking

Review the following social media posts and consider what risks you think the poster might be taking. What steps could they take to protect themselves better?

> "I'm soooo excited! We have just signed the contract for our new house. Moving in next weekend. Fingers crossed! Have a look at our fab new pad."
>
> Link to the estate details of the house (what you see is the colour photograph of the house, with the full address and post code, plus the floor plan)

Figure 2.2   Sample social media post (a).

> "Jim and I are looking forward to our short break in the Cotswolds this weekend. Kids are being packed off to Grandma's and the dog is at my sister's. They are all set to get pampered, so it's our turn for some pampering. 4 nights in this place!"
>
> Link to a nice hotel in the Cotswolds.

Figure 2.3   Sample social media post (b).

An outline answer is provided at the end of the chapter.

There are some common-sense approaches to using social media safely. Wherever possible, separate your personal and professional life by using different social media platforms for personal and professional use. If you identify yourself as a nursing associate, you must remain professional at all times, acting responsibly to uphold the reputation of the profession. Make sure your privacy settings are high and limit who can see what you post.

Do not accept friend requests or pursue relationships with either current or former patients, service users or their family members and friends. Never discuss work online; this includes conversations about or with patients and comments or complaints about colleagues, and do not post photographs. Remember, social media is not the place to air grievances or escalate a complaint, and everything you post online is public, even with the strictest privacy settings.

If you are not happy with a post appearing on the front page of a newspaper, don't post it.

Chapter summary

Adhering to the 4Ps of promoting professionalism and trust, preserving safety, prioritising people and practising effectively, as described by the NMC (2018a), we can ensure that we deliver effective, patient-centred, professional communication, which is the key to our success as healthcare professionals and for the safety of those in our care. We have explored how we use and share information and discussed the different processes we use, which includes considering the need to keep information confidential.

Through the exploration of handover excellence, there have been suggestions and trials for voice-recorded handovers and written/typed handover sheets which were printed and handed out to the nursing staff. Neither of these other methods were robust enough to ensure confidentiality. With the introduction of GDPR (2018), producing such materials would be in breach of these regulations because of inadequate security measures. We will explore this topic further in Chapter 3.

Significantly, we looked at the use of social media and have recognised that it is important to realise that even the strictest privacy settings have limitations. This is because once something is online, it can be copied and redistributed. Protect your professionalism and your reputation. If you are unsure whether something you post online could compromise your professionalism or your reputation, you should think about what the information means for you in practice and how it affects your responsibility to keep to the NMC *Code*.

Activities: Brief outline answers

Activity 2.2 Case study (page 30)

S	Situation Asking: What is going on with the patient?	An introduction (no need to do this if you are known to the listener): <ul><li>My name is (state your name)</li><li>I am a Nursing Associate on ward 5A</li></ul> **The reason for the communication** I would like to hand over this patient to you.
B	Background Asking: How did the patient come to be here?	Brief history: <ul><li>Mrs Choudhary is a 57-year-old lady who likes to be called Swarda.</li><li>She was admitted one week ago from A&E, following a two-week history of severe abdominal pain.</li><li>She had a total abdominal hysterectomy, and bilateral salpingo oophorectomy one week ago.</li></ul>

(Continued)

Figure 2.1a (Continued)

A	Assessment	Summary:
	Asking: What is the problem?	• ECG completed and no abnormalities detected • Urine output decreasing • Temperature increase • Pain controlled with patient-controlled analgesia • Bowels not open • IVI with fluid running. Dextrose and saline • Nasogastric tube (**Spigotted**) and nil by mouth • Wound oozing a lot • Robinson drain in place on the right-hand side • Her temperature has gone up and urine output down.
R	Recommendations	Plan:
	Asking: What is going to happen next for this patient?	• Regular observations • Check for bowel sounds and possibly encourage drinking and eating • Continue with intravenous fluids • Review wound and swab for infection • Physiotherapist recommends sitting her out in a chair and encourages deep breathing • Ensure the anti-embolism stocking continues to be worn • Consider antibiotics.
	Encourage questions and get listener to repeat key information to ensure it is understood.	

Figure 2.1a

Activity 2.3 Communication (page 31)

1.

- 57-year-old lady;
- one-day post operatively following total abdominal hysterectomy and bilateral salpingo oophorectomy;
- patient-controlled analgesia in place;
- Robinson wound drain in place on the right side of the wound;
- wound oozing a large amount of 'fluid';
- high temperature (pyrexia);
- an Electrocardiogram showed no abnormalities detected;
- urine output reduced, but has intravenous dextrose and saline fluids;
- nasogastric tube in place;
- bowels not opened;
- anti-embolism stocking worn.

2.

- 35-year-old man;
- admitted six days ago following a road traffic collision;

- fractured tibia and fibula in both legs;
- on 50% oxygen, respiratory rate of 25 breaths per minute;
- patient to be turned two-hourly;
- past medical history of asthma and needs nebulisers four times a day.

Activity 2.4 Case study: social media (page 32)

The NMC recommends not to make friend connections with patients either currently in your care or as ex-patients. How are you going to turn down an offer of friendship without hurting his or his parents' feelings while trying to maintain a caring and therapeutic relationship?

The first thing is not to reject the request before you see him, as he may feel rejected and have two days to dwell on a rejection before seeing you again.

Do not just ignore the request and pretend it didn't happen; it would end up feeling awkward.

The best course of action would be to talk to him about the request. Thank him for it and tell him that you are pleased he feels comfortable in your company and he respects you as a friend. You will, however, have to politely decline his request. As a professional nursing associate, you are bound by a code of ethics, and this does not allow you to form personal/friendship relationships with those you are caring or have cared for.

Be sure to make him understand this is not a rejection and it is nothing personal about him; it is just what is expected of you as a professional.

Activity 2.5 Critical thinking (page 34)

Think about how you would feel if you were the patient

I think it would be fair to say that you would feel vulnerable, betrayed and most likely scared. Having someone who you initially thought of as a trusted individual essentially become your stalker must make you terrified by such an invasion of your privacy. If she had a family, no doubt this fear would extend to protecting them. After all, if this nurse was prepared to breach their duty of care and act illegally, what else could they do?

What impact does the nurse's actions have on the hospital they worked in?

Certainly, for the individual this particular nurse had under observation, it would be easy to see how her trust in medical professionals would be severely affected. If the particulars about the stalking were printed in the local paper, or on social media, this would have ramifications for the hospital and the staff working in it. The public in general would quite rightly have concerns about the information they share and in trusting healthcare personnel in the hospital.

As nursing associates, you have an obligation to uphold the integrity of the profession.

Activity 2.6 Critical thinking (page 35)

"Devastated! The police have just left. Our house was broken into while we were away in the Cotswolds. Thankfully the kids can stay at Grandma's until we can get all this mess cleaned up. Police said it looked like they knew where to go, must have been stalking this place for weeks. So creepy when you think about it."

Figure 2.3a

By posting details like your address, or even a photo of yourself by your street's name, it gives people more information about yourself than you would rather share. So, be aware of your surroundings. Don't share plans in advance, if you can help it. Think about the pictures you post and how they would look out of context.

Knowledge review

Now that you have worked through the chapter, how would you rate your knowledge of the following topics?

		Good	Adequate	Poor
1.	the ways in which we share information			
2.	the correct use of the telephone and			
3.	verbal in-person handovers			
4.	the importance of note keeping			
5.	the dangers of social media			
6.	confidentiality			

If you are unsure of some aspects, what are you going to do next?

Further reading and useful websites

For NMC guidance on the responsible use of social media sites:
www.nmc.org.uk/globalassets/sitedocuments/nmc-publications/social-media-guidance.pdf

For more information on human rights and equality:
www.equalityhumanrights.com/en/human-rights-act/article-8-respect-your-private-and-family-life

For recent updates on reported drug names or appearance, read the government safety updates:
www.gov.uk/drug-safety-update/recent-drug-name-confusion

For more information on the Access to Medical Records Act (1990):
www.legislation.gov.uk/ukpga/1990/23/contents

For further information on GDPR (2018):
www.gov.uk/data-protection

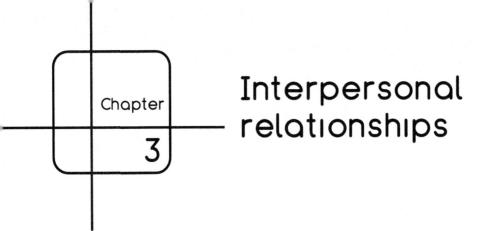

Chapter

3

Interpersonal relationships

Platform 4: Working in teams

At the point of registration, the nursing associate will be able to:

4.1   demonstrate an awareness of the roles, responsibilities and scope of practice of different members of the nursing and interdisciplinary team, and their own role within it.

Annexe A: Communication and relationship management skills

At the point of registration, the nursing associate will be able to safely demonstrate the following skills:

4.   Communication skills for working in professional teams:

Demonstrate effective skills when working in teams through:

4.1   active listening when receiving feedback and when dealing with team members' concerns and anxieties.
4.2   timely and appropriate escalation.
4.3   being a calm presence when exposed to situations involving conflict.
4.4   being assertive when required.

Chapter aims

By the end of this chapter, you will be able to:

- discuss NHS England's 6Cs and the NMC code.
- understand your personal values.
- understand the importance of self-awareness and how others perceive you.
- understand risks to patient safety and professional accountability
- discuss your role within the multidisciplinary team.

Introduction

Achieving success in your life through education, intellectual growth, forming healthy relationships and creating a community requires communication. Within the first two chapters, you have read about communication theory and have started to consider the nature of being a professional. This chapter is linked to Chapter 10 and is about introducing you to the dynamics of collaborative interprofessional team working. It focuses on behaviours, skills and attitudes linked to NHS England's (2012) 6Cs of compassionate care and the NMC *Code* (2018a) (see Figure 3.1). You will also be able to explore self-awareness, how your values and experiences inform the decisions you make and the way you respond to others.

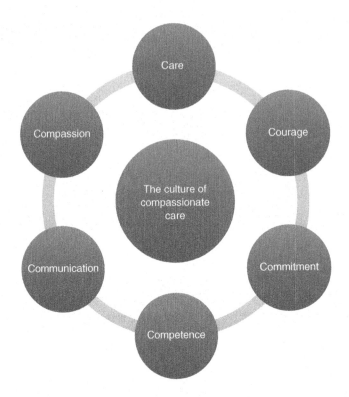

Figure 3.1   Defining the 6Cs.

Source: adapted from NHS England (2012)

In December 2012, the Chief Nursing Officer (CNO) for England, Jane Cummings, published the 6Cs, in conjunction with the CNOs of Wales and Scotland. For more information on the 6Cs strategy, go to the useful websites section at the end of this chapter.

The principles of the 6Cs are the core values of a national nursing strategy on compassion in practice. As a nursing associate, you are expected to strive towards applying the 6Cs in your practice. We will explore what each of the 6Cs mean and consider how they are used.

Courage

Courage is a crucial component of compassion. Courage allows us to do the right thing for the people in our care and gives us the opportunity to speak up when we feel something is not right. It also allows us to act as the advocate for those in our care and see how future actions may impact on the current care delivery, without consequences to our professionalism. Courage makes you resilient against difficult times and choices.

Compassion

Compassion literally means 'to suffer together' and is a feeling triggered by someone else's suffering. This feeling motivates you to want to help relieve the conditions that are causing the suffering state to the other person.

Compassion is central to therapeutic relationships and is described as intelligent kindness, which includes empathy, respect and dignity when providing care (NHS England, 2013).

Communication

Communication is crucial to a successful caring relationship and effective interprofessional working. As you have seen in the two previous chapters, there are various theories of communication and many ways in which we give and receive information. Communication is more than what we say and do. It is also about listening and making sure that the right people are involved in the communication to make it as effective as possible.

Commitment

As you have no doubt realised, becoming a nursing associate requires commitment and determination. Having that commitment to use your time, education and experience to improve services for those in your care and for the population that exists around you is an essential trait. Commitment requires resilience, particularly in challenging times such as those experienced in the Covid-19 pandemic. Despite the risks of contracting Covid-19, healthcare professionals kept working for the benefit of those in need of care. This is the embodiment of commitment.

Competence

Competence is the ability of combining all your knowledge, skills, values, attributes, beliefs and judgements, as well as your personal and professional behaviours, into action. The resulting action should be an educated act to provide effective and safe professional nursing care.

The NMC clearly dictates the values, experiences, skills and behaviour expected from a nursing associate. See the information about useful websites at the end of this chapter for more information on the NMC standard for nursing associates in section 13, where your personal accountability and level of competence is directly addressed.

Care

Care is central to your work and a core aspect of business within the profession. Caring defines you and people recognise this within you as a professional nursing associate.

Of all of the 6Cs, the act of caring is the most difficult to define, as there is no one way to do it. To care means to protect, to be concerned for, upkeep. 'Take care' can be a warning or an affectionate farewell. Care as defined for nursing associates is dependent on the environment and the needs of the individual or population you are employed to 'care for'. For you, caring is a matter of duty as outlined by the NMC and the expectations of your role.

You will be aware by now, having read the previous section, that the 6Cs are a collection of terms with meaning which must be used together, and no one single aspect of them can be used in isolation. Each of the Cs impacts on another one. For example, if you were working on a hospital ward which was dedicated to caring for patients with a Covid-19 positive status, you show courage and commitment even before you enter the ward before your shift. As the shift progresses, and you start work, you add caring, compassion, communication and competence into the list of what defines you and your duty as a nursing associate.

Activity 3.1 explores the 6Cs in action further.

Activity 3.1   Decision making: 6Cs

You are working in the emergency department in a local hospital, and you find yourself as part of a team of healthcare professionals, looking after a 26-year-old man who had been involved in a road traffic collision. The police arrive with the patient and are requesting that you get an urgent blood sample because they suspect he may be under the influence of alcohol.

The man is combative, confused and showing signs of a head injury with multiple facial lacerations that need attention. You try to put on a blood pressure cuff to start observations, but the patient hits out at you and pushes you away.

1.   Thinking of the 6Cs, what are your next steps at this point?

The police have noticed that a venous cannula has been inserted by the staff and they demand the urgent blood sample from you again.

2.   Thinking of the 6Cs, what are your next steps at this point?

Answers are proposed at the end of the chapter.

Having completed Activity 3.1, you will be able to recognise that there are situations that challenge your duty, and you will face a conflict of ideals. In the activity, you were challenged by the police, and as British citizens, you are brought up to respect the law and to assist the police, by default. We refer to this aspect of challenging professionals and accountability later on in this chapter.

The NMC Code and the 4Ps

In the most recent publication of *The Code: Professional Standards of Practice and Behaviours for Nurses, Midwives and Nursing Associates* (NMC, 2018a), a clear distinction of categories of expectations was made. These have come to be known as the 4Ps.

The role of the NMC is to set the standards in *The Code*, to which as a trainee and a registrant you must adhere. These are the standards that patients and members of the public expect from midwives, nurses and nursing associates. When joining the register and when renewing your registration as a nursing associate, you commit to upholding these standards and the expectations of an effective healthcare professional. The commitment to maintaining professional standards is fundamental to being part of a profession. Any failure to uphold the standards are taken very seriously and can result in you being removed from the register, so it is important that you understand what is expected of you.

The 4Ps form the section of the NMC *Code* and are to prioritise people, practise effectively, preserve safety and to promote professionalism and trust.

Prioritise people

You must put the interests of people using or needing healthcare services first. You make their care and safety your main concern and you must make sure that their dignity is preserved, and their needs are recognised, assessed and responded to. You must make sure that those receiving care are treated with respect, that their rights are upheld and that any discriminatory attitudes and behaviours towards those receiving care are challenged.

You know that people are central to your work as a nursing associate, and you may say 'of course we always put other people first'. You do need to be aware that it is not always that simple and there are challenges to putting people first.

For example, imagine that you are standing in the very middle of the ward you work on and two call bells alarm at the same time. The beds are the same distance away from you, but in different directions. You must choose which one to go to first. There is no way of knowing what the people who pressed the call bells need and neither person is any sicker or more at risk than the other.

It is a dilemma, and ultimately you will have to choose and put the needs of one person over and above the other one. There is no right answer to this, but as long as your intention is not to cause harm or to deprive anyone of healthcare services, whatever decision you make in this instance is defendable.

Practise effectively

You should assess need and deliver or advise on treatment or give help (including preventative or rehabilitative care) without too much delay and to the best of your abilities, on the basis of best available evidence. You must communicate effectively and keep clear and accurate records. You should share skills, knowledge and experience, where appropriate. You should also reflect and act on any feedback you receive to improve your practice.

If you were to ask most healthcare professionals, they would define practising effectively as a good clinical outcome or a procedure well performed. The NMC are clear that *The Code* contains the standards that patients and members of the public expect from health professionals. So, a patient may have a set of different expectations of effective practice. It is important to try and see effectiveness from the patient's perspective. One obvious expectation would be that the care you are delivering is up to date, educated and informed. In essence, this P emphasises the need for continuous professional development (CPD).

Preserve safety

You must make sure that patients' and public safety is not affected. You must work within the limits of your competence, exercising your professional 'duty of candour' and raising concerns immediately whenever you come across situations that put patients' or public safety at risk. You must take necessary action to deal with any concerns where appropriate.

Safety is a huge topic which has had much attention over recent years. Martin et al. (2019) state that adverse events which result in unintentional harm or injury affect between 3% and 23% of patients, with 3.6% resulting in avoidable deaths in hospital. It was the reports of unusually high rates of unnecessary deaths that highlighted the failures at the Mid Staffordshire NHS Foundation Trust which prompted the Francis Report of 2013, which investigated the failures in the trust.

The Francis Report tells you that there are certain aspects that impact on patient safety. It is clear that patient safety coincides with patient-centred care and the combining factors surrounding care provision. The Berwick Report (Berwick, 2013) also shows us that much more can be done to address safety when we unite.

The four key aims from this report are:

- placing the quality of patient care, especially patient safety, above all other aims;
- engaging, empowering and hearing patients and carers at all times;
- fostering whole-heartedly the growth and development of all staff, including their ability and support to improve the processes in which they work;
- embracing transparency unequivocally and everywhere, in the service of accountability, trust and the growth of knowledge.

Consider the elements of safety in the scenario in Activity 3.2.

Activity 3.2   Critical thinking: safety

It is midweek at 12:30 on a busy 28-bedded elderly medical ward and the following four situations have arisen at the same time.

- The charge nurse is off the ward for a departmental meeting, leaving a less experienced band 6 senior staff nurse in charge.
- The ward cleaner had just finished cleaning the floor in the corridor and decided to take her break, off the unit. Unfortunately, the cleaner had forgotten to place the wet floor warning sign in the corridor.
- The cleaner joined three of the six ward staff who had just been sent on their break.
- Mrs Garcia, an elderly patient who is in a confused state with mobility issues, has been walking the ward. In that moment, she thinks that her name has been called from the corridor.

What possible risks can you foresee in this situation?

At 12:45, Mrs Garcia, in her confused state, decided to respond to the voice she heard and tried to find the source. Mrs Garcia forgot the need for shoes and her mobility aid.

So, in her stockinged feet, she entered the corridor and slipped on the wet floor, falling on her hip.

At 12:55, the band 6 senior staff nurse who had been left in charge managed to get Mrs Garcia back to bed. She didn't want to look bad in front of the charge nurse or be punished by the hospital for having to report an unobserved fall, so she does not follow hospital policy and does not complete the appropriate accident report form or get a doctor to see Mrs Garcia.

Mrs Garcia's safety had been compromised; can you identify the following failures?

Human failure:

Management failure:

Organisational failure:

Answers can be found at the end of the chapter.

Reflecting on Activity 3.2, you can see that there is no simple cause of the incident to Mrs Garcia; rather, it is a combination of factors in a sequence. It would be useful for you to think of a combination of factors that you have experienced that have led to some harm or a near miss.

It is also important to recognise the factors which the culture in the workplace have on patient safety, as identified by the Francis Report (2013). The Francis Report was published because of safety failings at the Mid Staffordshire NHS Foundation Trust. The report found that:

- there was a culture of bullying;
- priorities were target driven and not patient centred;
- there was a disengagement from management;
- there was low staff morale;
- there was a culture of isolation between departments and staff;
- there was a lack of **candour** or honesty between staff;
- there was a culture of acceptance of or **apathy** towards poor behaviours;
- there was a culture of denial among staff.

(Entwistle, 2013)

In response to reports such as the Francis Report, a number of tools have been developed specifically to help healthcare workers promote patient safety. An example of this is the National Early Warning Signs (NEWS) tool, which is designed to help staff to identify early signs of deterioration in the patient's condition and that urgent attention may be required (RCN, 2020b).

Regardless of the development of helpful tools to promote safety, the real key to safety is you. Thinking back to Activities 3.1 and 3.2, in conjunction with the list of safety failings found following the Mid Staffordshire NHS Foundation Trust investigation, we can see that the human factor is central to harm prevention and the choices you make as practitioners. It also underlines the need for courage as one of the 6Cs.

Promote professionalism and trust

You must always uphold the reputation of your profession. You should display a personal commitment to the standards of practice and behaviour set out in *The Code*. You should be a model of integrity and leadership for others to aspire to. This should lead to trust and confidence in the professions from patients, people receiving care, other health and care professionals and the public.

Being a professional nursing associate is much more than wearing a uniform and a name badge. Although the uniform is a symbol of a professional, there is much more to it; it carries great privilege and responsibility. As a nursing associate with compassion, which as you will recall means to 'suffer with', you will get to experience life-changing events. Being present at the birth of a child, hearing the announcement that their cancer is in remission, or the death of a loved one is a privileged position to be in. To have this opportunity is not to be squandered and disrespected, as you will see people at their most vulnerable and you must be trustworthy, act with integrity and supply a high standard of individualised patient-centred care.

Personal values

To honestly perform as a professional nursing associate, you must be aware of your personal values and have the ability of self-reflection. You will know that negotiating a clear and direct path between the challenges you will face in the course of your work and your duty of care can be difficult. The difficulty is eased when you work as a cohesive team with shared core values, and you are aware of your intrapersonal communication.

Intra, meaning within, focuses on that inner voice or the things that make you who you are. Intrapersonal communication focuses on the self-concept or self-awareness. This is about knowing what you are feeling and why you are feeling it, the collection of your personal values, beliefs and attitudes that determines how you think about yourself and how you engage with others. It also guides you and acts as a 'moral compass'.

Aspects such as body image and self-esteem are intertwined with the self-concept and are a means of seeing yourself as others may see you, in relation to societal or cultural norms. They are dependent on past encounters and experiences which may be negative or positive (McKinnon, 2016).

It is essential that you get to know yourself and explore your perception, which is the outward-facing mind experiencing the world. This is still firmly connected with the values, beliefs and attitudes that make up the self-concept. Being aware of this is essential for developing self-awareness and the ability to reflect, as this increases resilience (Luft and Ingham, 1955).

Identifying and understanding your values is a challenging and important exercise. Your personal values are a central part of who you are and who you want to be. By becoming more aware of these important factors in your life, you can use them as a guide to make the best choice in any situation.

Some of life's decisions are really about determining what you value most. When many options seem reasonable, it is helpful and comforting to rely on your values and use them as a strong guiding force to point you in the right direction. Activity 3.3 asks you to explore your personal values and place them in order of importance.

Activity 3.3   Reflection: prioritise your top ten personal values

Exploring your personal values is difficult, because you will have to look deep inside yourself. It is also extremely important because, when making a decision, you will have to choose between solutions that may satisfy different values. This is when you must know which value is more important to you.

Write down your top ten values, in no particular order. Some examples of a personal value could be:

Proud Caring Energetic Happy Shy Independent

Please see the end of the chapter for more examples of adjectives which could define your values.

Look at your first two values and ask yourself, 'If I could satisfy only one of these, which would I choose?' It might help to visualise a situation in which you would have to make that choice. For example, if you compare the values of service and stability, imagine that you must decide whether to sell your house and move to another country to do valuable foreign aid work, or keep your house and volunteer to do charity work closer to home.

Keep working through the list, by comparing each value with each other value, until your list is in the correct order with your strongest personal value at the top.

Make a note of the top three: these are your default core values.

There is a list of suggested values to help you at the end of this chapter.

In Activity 3.3, you generated a list of your personal inner values. These inner thoughts and feelings go some way to defining your core values. Before you express anything, you need to address the intrapersonal communication before you can address the interpersonal.

You need to explore your perception, which is the outward-facing mind experiencing the world. This is still very firmly connected with the values, beliefs and attitudes which make up the self-concept.

Johari window model of self

During this chapter, you have been getting to know yourself. We will now be exploring how others see you. Luft and Ingham (1955), as cited by McKinnon (2016), developed a commonly used model used for training and helping people understand self-awareness, personal development for the purpose of improving communication, interpersonal development and team development.

The Johari window uses four perspectives or quadrants, as they are defined in the model. These four quadrants represent information about feelings, experiences, views, attitudes, skills and intentions about a person in relation to their group.

In Activity 3.4, you are asked to explore the perception of other people on the self that is you, using the Johari window.

Activity 3.4   Critical thinking: Johari window

Choose a colleague(s) with whom to complete this activity. Using the core values that you identified in Activity 3.3 and using the list of adjectives at the end of this chapter, with your colleague(s), complete the activity. Please draw your own blank grid, based on the one below.

Look at the grid below and the examples within the boxes (see Figure 3.2).

1. Of the ten values you have previously identified in Activity 3.3, pick the top eight.
2. Your colleague(s) will also pick their top eight from the list at the end of the chapter that they think best describes you.
3. Each of you will reveal the eight adjectives that best describe you.
4. Check these against your list and write them in the Johari window as follows:
   a. If your colleague(s) has chosen an adjective that you had also chosen, then write this in the open area or arena box.
   b. If your colleague(s) has chosen an adjective which is not on your list, then this goes in the blind spot box.
   c. Anything left from your list should be written in the hidden area or facade box.
   d. Everything else on the list of 56 adjectives which have not been chosen by either yourself or the colleague(s) are unknown.

	Known to self	Not known to self
Known to others	**Open area or Arena** Your top eight core values should be listed here. These are the values identified in Activity 3.3. These are the values known to you and seen by others. It is a person's most prevalent or obvious characteristics. *Example: "Everyone knows that I am dependable, because I am always on time."*	**Blind spot** The values selected for you by a friend or colleague. The attributes that others selected for you, but you did not select for yourself. Subconscious characteristics, or external perceptions that you don't identify with. *Example: "I didn't know that I am seen as being bold."*
Not known to others	**Hidden area or Facade** The attributes that you selected but others didn't select for you. These are characteristics that are not externally present or obvious. *Example: "I feel like I am independent, but I don't share that";"You don't see that I am independent?"*	**Unknown** The rest: attributes that neither you nor others selected for you. These are irrelevant characteristics. *Example:"I'm not spontaneous."*

Figure 3.2   Johari window activity.

Reflect on this activity, and consider the following questions:

1. What were the biggest surprises to you regarding the blind spots?
2. Which adjectives are helpful to you to know from what the others had picked?
3. What hidden adjectives would you like to show more often to your team colleagues?

As this is a personal and subjective activity, there is no model answer.

Activity 3.4 has allowed you to explore how you feel you represent yourself, but also how others perceive you. It is a valuable exercise which allows you to make sense of the image and adjectives you project and the differences between what you think you project and what others perceive.

Having understood the intrapersonal, we can look closely at what it means to be a professional in an interpersonal team. Being part of a healthcare team not only means that you need to be educated and knowledgeable, but you are required to have strong interpersonal skills too.

You must be able to communicate and use a wide range of communication techniques, as seen in Chapter 1.

Interpersonal skills are the tools people use to interact with and communicate with individuals in an organisational environment. There are nine main areas of interpersonal communication that we need to consider:

- verbal communication;
- non-verbal communication;
- listening skills;
- negotiation;
- problem solving;
- decision making;
- assertiveness;
- patience;
- empathy.

In Activity 3.5, you will need to think about ways in which you communicate, using some of the interpersonal communications skills listed above.

Activity 3.5   Communication

No one is perfect when it comes to communication, and just about everyone can do better and become more effective. Effective communication is essential for your role as a nursing associate and is something you should strive towards practising and improving. Take this short quiz to identify your communication strengths and weaknesses.

(Continued)

(Continued)

1. I demonstrate that I am listening by nodding or saying words and phrases like, 'Yes,' 'I see' and 'Uh huh':
   a. always/almost always
   b. often
   c. sometimes
   d. rarely/never

2. I can read another person's mood by watching their body language and facial expressions:
   a. always/almost always
   b. often
   c. sometimes
   d. rarely/never

3. I maintain eye contact with the person I'm conversing with at all times:
   a. always/almost always
   b. often
   c. sometimes
   d. rarely/never

4. When having to deliver correction or criticism to someone (e.g. a child, significant other or employee), I stay focused on identifying the problem and seeking a solution rather than shouting:
   a. always/almost always
   b. often
   c. sometimes
   d. rarely/never

5. I treat others respectfully even when I strongly disagree or they have upset me:
   a. always/almost always
   b. often
   c. sometimes
   d. rarely/never

6. I refrain from using absolutes like 'always' and 'never' when having a disagreement or argument with someone (e.g. 'I'm always the one who has to fix things' or 'You never care about my feelings'):
   a. always/almost always
   b. often
   c. sometimes
   d. rarely/never

7. I try to avoid spreading or participating in gossip:
   a. always/almost always
   b. often
   c. sometimes
   d. rarely/never

8. If I think I know what someone is going to say, I finish their sentences for them:

   a. always/almost always
   b. often
   c. sometimes
   d. rarely/never

9. I'm quick to offer solutions when someone is telling me about their problems:

   a. always/almost always
   b. often
   c. sometimes
   d. rarely/never

10. I try to think of a good or clever response while the other person is still speaking:

    a. always/almost always
    b. often
    c. sometimes
    d. rarely/never

11. I try to use fancy vocabulary words and jargon so that people know I am intelligent:

    a. always/almost always
    b. often
    c. sometimes
    d. rarely/never

12. I try to have the last word in any conversation or discussion:

    a. always/almost always
    b. often
    c. sometimes
    d. rarely/never

Analysis of your answers can be found at the end of the chapter.

In Activity 3.5, you have been able to explore your interprofessional communication traits and have been able to identify a couple of areas that may need improvement or refining. Make a plan to re-look at Activity 3.5 once you have completed Chapter 6 and then compare your results. Hopefully, this will demonstrate some improvements.

Precise communication

In the first instance, you must possess the ability to actively listen to patients when they are describing their symptoms. To actively listen is to make a conscious effort to hear and pay attention to what a person is telling you. This is not just the words they use, but the complete message being communicated. You have to remember that your average patient will not be familiar with medical terminology, and they may not be able to express what they are feeling in any kind of symptoms diagnosis (Levitt, 2001).

Within your role as the nursing associate, you must listen carefully and try to decode the clues to the symptoms. Verbally repeating this to the patient for confirmation or correction is good practice to ensure you have heard them accurately. You cannot allow yourself to become distracted and must not interrupt the person as they try to communicate with you.

The next phase is to establish the priority of this information and escalate the communication to whoever is best suited to address the patient's needs in a timely manner.

The accurate relaying of this information is the vital next step. A useful tool for this is the SBAR communication tool – Situation, Background, Assessment, Recommendation.

As seen in Chapter 2, SBAR is an easy to use, structured form of communication that enables information to be transferred accurately between individuals. It consists of standardised prompt questions in four sections to ensure that you are sharing concise and focused information. It allows you to communicate assertively and effectively, reducing the need for repetition and the likelihood for errors. As the structure is shared, it also helps you anticipate the information needed by colleagues and encourages assessment skills (ACT Academic, 2018).

Patience, empathy and humour

Establishing communication with a patient often requires patience, and effective healthcare team members should provide information that calms an upset family or team member without leaving them feeling anxious or agitated. With an upset patient, you could seek to reassure them and put them at ease with some appropriate and gentle humour. Appropriately used humour can lighten a tense atmosphere and may raise depressed spirits. The ability to use humour should not be underestimated, and healthcare professionals with this skill have frequently been able to maintain peaceful, cooperative relationships with patients and their families.

As much as humour can be an outlet for stress and tension, the emphasis here though is on appropriately used humour, as there will be many times when the seriousness of a situation requires nothing less than a serious and a professional approach.

Team identity

Having a strong team identity equates to effective interpersonal communication. This, in turn, has a positive impact on organisational skills, performance and overall job satisfaction.

Lessons learned from the Francis Report (2013) identified that there are many factors that come together to cause the circumstances that immediate healthcare teams cannot control. What you can control is the working on building a team that provides support and encouragement. Healthcare teams who work well together promote higher morale, lower stress levels and they maintain safer environments for patients and peers. The development of positive and effective teams will be explored in more depth in Chapter 10.

Conflict resolution and decision making

Confliction in the workplace should not be about hostility and arguing; it is the exploration of conflicting points of view. When managed properly, and where effective communication is present, any conflict or disagreement should not dissolve into disharmony and can be used as a learning opportunity.

Conflicts that cause disruption are when one party/body of people seeks to defeat and undermine the other party/body. Often, conflicts like this are caused when resources are stretched and responsibilities are compromised. I am sure you can all relate to staff shortages and how this impacts on your ability to cope and your temperament. This discussion of conflict and conflict resolution is explored in more depth in Chapter 5.

Those healthcare professionals who can set aside their emotions and recognise them objectively are best placed to see the conflict from both sides. This ability usually coincides with a genuine desire to find a resolution to a conflict. Confronting and resolving issues in a mature and professional manner is an indication of emotional maturity. It is important that all healthcare professionals, including nursing associates, use logic, evidence-based education and self-reflection to make critical workplace decisions. The topic of emotional intelligence and how you manage your emotions in conflict situations will be explored in more depth in Chapter 6.

Promoting positive communication patterns and assertiveness

All healthcare professionals and nursing associates are no different in that to do your job effectively, you need to be in possession of all the relevant facts and explanations about activities affecting your care delivery. It may be necessary to put your emotions aside and question a team member about their rationale behind a care decision. This ensures that the information you have is accurate, which helps you in maintaining positive relationships with patients and peers as well as reducing miscommunications and confusion.

Assertiveness, and the confidence and courage to ask intelligent questions, in the workplace promotes an environment that cultivates teamwork, understanding, trust and mutual respect.

Chapter summary

This chapter explored the 6Cs and the 4Ps in relation to communication and good practice. Throughout this chapter, we have focused on your values and self-awareness and how we should perform and how we are viewed by others and, by default, by the wider interprofessional team.

We have seen that this is a clear rationale for the NHS improvements relevant to communication and the direct links to patient safety. Within this aspect, we have explored your communication effectiveness and clearly outlined the correct engagement with communication and the interprofessional team.

Activities: Brief outline answers

Activity 3.1 Decision making: 6Cs (page 44)

1. What are your next steps here?

The next step is to summon *courage* and reaffirm your *commitment* to caring and approach the patient again in order to secure the blood pressure cuff. You could also *communicate* with another member of the team to help you.

2. What are your next steps here?

Using *courage* again, you must tell the police to wait. Firstly, in terms of being *competent*, you, as nursing associate, are not qualified to take blood from a venous cannula, and so will not get them a blood sample from the cannula. Secondly, with *compassion*, the patient lacks capacity at this stage, and he cannot give his consent for his blood to be taken, so you must work in his best interests and *care* for his immediate health needs, which must take priority.

It is important to have the courage to challenge authority and be an advocate for your patient. The police do not have the right to request blood from an unconscious patient; however, they can make a request to the doctor in charge. It is then the doctor's decision whether blood can be taken from the patient.

After the patient has had their immediate care needs addressed and is stable, you could decide to complete an incident form for an injury incurred during the patient's agitated state when they pushed you away.

Activity 3.2 Critical thinking: safety (page 46)

What possible risks can you foresee in this situation?

*   With the charge nurse off the ward, a less experienced staff member was left in charge. She sent three of the ward staff on break at the same time, leaving the ward understaffed and unsafe.
*   The ward cleaner had just finished mopping the floor, so the floor is likely to be wet. With no warning sign, there is a risk of slipping.
*   With three of the ward staff on their break, there was no one around to remind Mrs Garcia to wear her shoes and to use her walking frame. No one was able to recognise the risk of the wet floor.

Mrs Garcia's safety had been compromised. Can you identify the following failures?

*   Human failure: the ward cleaner's forgetfulness and the staff nurse wilfully ignoring hospital protocols.
*   Management failure: the decision to allow three nursing staff to go on break at the same time left the ward with insufficient staff to ensure patients' safety.

- Organisational failure: the hospital's culture of punishing staff for mistakes, rather than seeing each accident or mistake as an opportunity for learning that could improve services throughout the hospital, acted as a strong disincentive for the staff nurse to follow standard protocols and seek urgent medical assistance for Mrs Garcia.

Activity 3.3 Reflection (page 49)

Prioritise your top ten personal values			
Able	Energetic	Loving	Searching
Accepting	Extroverted	Mature	Self-assertive
Adaptable	Friendly	Modest	Self-conscious
Bold	Giving	Nervous	Sensible
Brave	Happy	Observant	Sentimental
Calm	Helpful	Organised	Shy
Caring	Idealistic	Patient	Silly
Cheerful	Independent	Powerful	Spontaneous
Clever	Ingenious	Proud	Sympathetic
Complex	Intelligent	Quiet	Tense
Confident	Introverted	Reflective	Trustworthy
Dependable	Kind	Relaxed	Warm
Dignified	Knowledgeable	Religious	Wise
Empathetic	Logical	Responsive	Witty

Figure 3.3 Example values.

Activity 3.5 Communication (page 51)

The first six questions reflect effective communication skills. So, if you answered 'always/almost always' or 'often', you are heading in the right direction and are developing appropriate communication skills. Your listening skills, speaking habits and emotional intelligence are above average.

If you found the third question difficult to answer, you are right to stop and think about this answer. In some cultures, eye contact can cause offence, and the person you are talking to may also feel embarrassed and may not want to meet your eye. Keeping a balance of the right amount of eye contact is a difficult skill to master, so practise.

If you answered 'sometimes' or 'rarely/never', your skills need some practice and reflection. With practice, over time and with good supportive feedback, good communication skills can be learned and developed.

The last five questions reflect negative habits and traits. If you answered 'sometimes' or 'rarely/never', you are aware of appropriate professional interactions. You demonstrate maturity and wisdom in communicating with others.

If you answered 'always/almost always' or 'often', then there is room for improvement. Any step towards improvement means identifying your weakness. You might want to consider marking an action plan with the SMART (specific, measurable, achievable, realistic and timed) goals.

Knowledge review

Now that you have worked through the chapter, how would you rate your knowledge of the following topics?

	Good	Adequate	Poor
• NHS England's 6Cs and the NMC *Code*			
• your personal values			
• the importance of self-awareness and how others perceive you			
• risks to patient safety and professional accountability			
• your role within the multidisciplinary team			

If you are unsure of some aspects, what are you going to do next?

Further reading and useful websites

For further information on the 6Cs, visit the NHS England website:
www.england.nhs.uk/6cs/wp-content/uploads/sites/25/2015/03/introducing-the-6cs.pdf

For more information on the rights of a patient under your care being investigated by the police following a road traffic collision:
www.legislation.gov.uk/ukpga/1988/52/contents

The Francis Report was published on 6 February 2013 and examined the causes of the failings in care at Mid Staffordshire NHS Foundation Trust between 2005 and 2009:
www.health.org.uk/responding-to-the-francis-inquiry-report

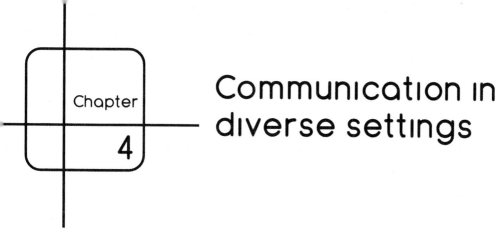

Communication in diverse settings

Chapter aims

By the end of this chapter, you will be able to:

- differentiate between the four fields of nursing.
- describe some of the settings where nursing takes place.
- understand some of the factors that help achieve effective communication.
- describe barriers to communication by setting.
- understand whom institutional theory can impact on communication.

Introduction

As you know, nursing is amazingly diverse and, as a generic role, the nursing associate is arguably the most varied of all the healthcare professional roles. A nursing associate is not bound to stick within one of the four fields of nursing (Mental Health, Learning Disability, Adult or Child). This could be seen as a challenge or a gift. You might argue that having knowledge of a wide range of nursing fields and specialisms gives you more scope of practice. Certainly, the government and the NMC see the role of the trained nursing associate as a valuable team member with a more generalist knowledge. In this chapter, you will explore the diverse settings where healthcare activities take place.

In whatever area you work in, it is important to take time to understand the social structure, the rules (written and unwritten), the norms and routines for social behaviour. One common example is the use of the term 'service user' rather than 'patient' in mental health settings. These rules and norms are referred to as the institutional theory of an environment. Understanding the institutional theory will help you understand the challenges faced by the patients and the other staff. Instructional theory looks at the social structure of the environment and asks you:

What are rules?

What are the norms and routines?

Who is the authority?

Understanding these will help you establish the guidelines for social behaviour (Crew and Levins, 2019). Understanding the social rules will help focus your communication appropriately and give you a clear structure to follow.

General hospitals and acute care - in hospital

General hospitals vary in size and are categorised by the number of beds. Large general hospitals will have over 500 beds and are usually situated in cities. These are often associated closely with a local university, such as Queen's Medical Centre in Nottingham, which has 1,300 beds. A medium general hospital will typically have between 100 and 499 beds and be found in towns with smaller populations, such as the Great Western Hospital in Swindon, Wiltshire, with 480 beds. A small general hospital will have less than 100 beds and will be found in smaller towns. These are often part of a larger hospital trust, such as Newark Hospital in Nottinghamshire with its 36 beds. This hospital is allied to the Sherwood Forest Hospitals NHS Foundation Trust which has four hospitals of varying sizes and specialisms.

These are general hospitals in the sense that they admit all types of medical and surgical cases. The larger the hospital, the more services can be offered, although they all focus on acute illnesses which require relatively short-term care.

Acute care can be defined as secondary healthcare. It is where a patient will receive active, short-term treatment for an injury or an episode of illness that cannot be suitably treated in the community or at home. Acute care is also for emergency medical treatment and for invasive surgical procedures and the initial recovery period. Acute care can be the use of diagnostic services, such as x-ray, and may require follow-up with an outpatient clinic, or it can be for a condition requiring a hospital stay, as for an inpatient.

Specialist hospitals

Specialist hospitals are like general hospitals in the sense that they have the same general structure and will have similarities in the equipment used to diagnose and treat patients. These hospitals are a tertiary service with a particular role, so instead of them taking all manner of general conditions, they are focused on very specific problems or conditions.

Examples of specialist hospitals are:

Hospital for Tropical Diseases

Great Ormond Street Hospital (care of children and adolescents)

Goodmayes Hospital (mental health facility)

Bristol Eye Hospital

Royal National Orthopaedic Hospital (RNOH)

Western Park Hospital (which specialises in cancer treatment)

Harefield Hospital (specialises in heart and lung)

Broadmoor Hospital (psychiatric specialism)

Michael Rutter Centre for Children and Adolescents (for children living with mental illness, specifically anorexia)

Inpatient

Being an inpatient requires an overnight stay in a hospital for at least one night. During this time, they are under the care and supervision of a nurse, nursing associate, doctor and/or midwife. In terms of institutional theory, this is more acutely seen with the patients themselves. They fall into a sick role (Bass and Halligan, 2014) where they take on behaviours they believe are expected for a hospital environment.

When a patient is admitted to hospital, it is an anxious time for them and their close family and friends. They often struggle to anticipate what is going to happen to them and how they are going to feel. As nursing associates whose workplace is the inpatient environment, it is easy for you to 'feel at home' in the inpatient environment. For the patient, however, this is an alien place where they don't know the rules and what is socially acceptable. This would be particularly applicable for those in distress from pain or anxiety, but also with people living with a mental health condition or a condition which requires order and routine. We will explore how this would feel in Activity 4.1.

Activity 4.1   Reflection

Imagine an occasion when you have felt socially awkward at a gathering of people you do not know. Maybe you are in a situation where you did not speak the language and you needed help from someone to whom you could not talk in a familiar language, or you found yourself on an unfamiliar public transport system with no map and no money.

How did you feel in this situation when you had someone familiar with you?

How did those feelings differ from when you were on your own?

How are you going to know you are not offending someone or making a fool of yourself?

These answers are subjective and individual to you, so there is no model answer.

From Activity 4.1, it is easy see that being with someone familiar in a challenging situation makes you feel better, but once you are on your own, you may feel panic and apprehension. Once visiting time is over and the patient is alone, navigating the unfamiliar environment is increasingly difficult. You are using jargon and words they do not understand, which is not unlike speaking an unfamiliar language. There is no handbook for patient conduct and each clinical environment has its own quirks, which makes a hospital a confusing and scary place, not unlike finding yourself on a strange public transport system with no map and no money. We recognise the importance of communication and the stress this can induce if we get it wrong. Some of the aspects we cannot control, but much of it we can when we take time to consider and reflect on how we communicate.

Outpatient clinic or outpatient surgery

This is when a person attends the hospital for treatment or diagnosis, without the need to stay in the hospital overnight. This is the preferable option for most people, as they get to recover comfortably in their own home in familiar surroundings. It also reduces, but does not eliminate, the risks of the patient contracting a hospital-acquired infection (Hefzy et al., 2016).

Communication in this environment is focused on instructions and managing expectations, which shares similarities with consultations in a general practice (GP) surgery, where time is very tight. We will explore some of the challenges of communication in clinics in Chapter 5.

Urgent or emergency care

The high-stress, high-risk environment of an emergency department can mean that effective communication is compromised.

The highly skilled team will focus on clinical aspects of the trauma, as the priority and the roles of the clinical staff will be clearly communicated. The quicker treatment is started after a traumatic injury, the more likely it is that the patient will survive. This initial period is often referred to as the 'golden hour' (Pham et al., 2017). From the chaos and pain of sudden traumatic injury, a patient will experience rapid changes in environment, temperature and sounds. They stop in an unfamiliar room under bright lights, where they are surrounded by strangers in masks who will strip them, take their blood, put in needles and move them around to poke and examine. While the strangers shout instructions and orders to each other, they are in pain and trying to make sense of what is going on. It sounds like a story line from a horror film, but it is a reasonable account of an emergency admission. Kaufman (2017) explored how some patients felt about their experience in a trauma centre and summarised his findings.

Kaufman also established that some thought the communication was clear, whereas others were concerned and confused by what was happening and the nature of their injuries. Introductions and explanations were brief, and some patients reported that they thought the practitioners were talking negatively about them out of their ear shot. Most of the participants expressed concerns about work and their family which were not shared with the staff, which added to their anxiety.

Many of those interviewed recalled having their clothes cut off. This acted as a signal to the seriousness of the situation. Some expressed upset about the damage and loss of their clothes.

If communication with the patient in the moment is not possible or practical due to the nature of the trauma, a debrief of the events could be a useful alternative to address any remaining confusion or anxiety for the patient. This is called Critical Incident Stress Debriefing (CISD).

The first step with CISD would be to let the patient know that you care and that you are there to offer emotional or practical help and support. It is not usual that a person who has been through a trauma will appear withdrawn, emotionally numb or over stimulated. Whatever their emotional state or needs are, it is important that they know you are there for them if and when they need you to be. The next action, and the longer-term step, is to highlight resources, such as counselling and mental health services that they may consider using (Navarro et al., 2021).

If embarking on a debrief for staff after a traumatic event, the element of reflection is key. A useful tool in team debriefing is the TALK guide. The guide is supportive and includes structures for conversations about an event, which does not focus on the negatives but allows for effective and constructive communication that creates a solution-based strategy (Navarro et al., 2021).

Community-based

There are several services that can be considered close to home. These include the following:

- outreach services;
- dialysis centres;
- rehab centres;
- hospices.

There will be others that are specific to your location and will be linked to a local charity, so the list above is by no means exhaustive. This section will be looking at the services that are universal and are familiar to every region.

General practitioner surgery

GP provision is the starting place for the vast majority of clinical conditions and diagnosis. Data from the Office of National Statistics in 2018 stated that there are 7,051 GP surgeries serving in the community across the United Kingdom. This number of surgeries is decreasing year by year and is expected to continue to decline due to the underfunding of the primary care service (British Medical Association, 2020).

As of October 2018, there were 59,416,013 patients registered with a GP, which equates to 91.3% of the population. This leaves approximately 5.6 million people within the UK without a GP. In the same month, there were 29.6 million GP appointments made, which equates to 45% of the total population. If we make a broad assumption that all the GP surgeries are the same size (we know they are not), each surgery will see 4,209 patients a month.

With this little bit of perspective on the status of primary care, we can now think about communication. The average time for a Practice Nurse's appointment in a GP surgery is between 10 and 15 minutes, which is less time than it would take to make the appointment in the first place.

In some cases, a 15-minute appointment is ample time to discuss a problem and get a solution and for the patient to leave satisfied. However, there is increasing pressure on primary care due to:

- an ageing population with multiple co-morbidities;
- redirection of care from secondary service to primary care;
- increased patient expectations;
- the extended role of the nurse and nursing associate.

Often, those patients with multiple conditions and complex and time-consuming psychosocial issues are required to make multiple appointments.

Ten- to fifteen-minute consultations are also stressful for staff because, the more complex the consultation, the more time you need to spend on documenting the communication. Then the next patient comes in with a different set of problems for discussion, which you need to focus on. You will need to be able to adapt seamlessly between seeing patients of all ages, conditions and capacity levels.

It is clear to see that there are challenges in communicating in general practice due to external pressures, but it can also be very rewarding because you build professional caring relationships with your patients.

The real skill in successful communication in this environment is being able to start each consultation as a brand-new event, entirely focused on the patient you are with. If their appointment has been delayed and they have had to wait, you should apologise for their wait. Your communication must be professional and succinct. Once you have the facts at your disposal or have done some clinical measurements, you will be ready to discuss the options. You must then ask the patient if they are happy with the plan/treatments and if they have any questions. You should round up the consultation quickly and professionally, write your notes and move on to the next new encounter. We shall explore the difficult consultation more in Activity 4.2.

Activity 4.2   Work-based learning

In your role as a nursing associate in general practice, there can be some challenging situations, which often involve children.

The scenario is that you are running a baby immunisation clinic and baby Archie Station is eight weeks old and due for his first immunisations. Archie's paternal grandfather brings him to the appointment for his vaccinations. The grandfather says he volunteered to bring Archie because Archie's mother would get all upset. He also says that they have discussed it as a family and they don't want baby Archie to have a polio injection. They want it as the drop on sugar cube like they used to do it.

As the nursing associate in this position, what are you going to do here?

Suggested answers are available at the end of the chapter.

Activity 4.2 shows how a relatively simple issue of consent can get very complicated. Having the ability to find the answers to unexpected questions or situations out of the norm is an important skill to develop.

Telehealth/video health calls and remote access to healthcare

Communicating via telehealth is the use of electronic information and telecommunication. The purpose is to support long-distance health needs and to widen the availability of accessing the healthcare services that you need.

According to the World Health Organisation (WHO), telehealth is the delivery of healthcare services where distance or remoteness is a factor. Healthcare professionals engage in telehealth using a range of communication technologies that allow for the exchange of information regarding diagnosis, treatments, and preventions of injuries and diseases. Telehealth can also be used for research, education and the evaluation of care and services (WHO, 2010).

Communicating remotely, such as via a telephone, means that you lose some of the skills associated with effective communication. For example, you will not be able to see the patients' faces or assess their body language. You will not be able to provide therapeutic touch and cannot assess their environment for danger. A clear benefit of mobile technology is the ability for it to be automatically traced, which helps determine the location of the call.

It can be a problem in telehealth to obtain accurate and meaningful information on the patient's condition. The level of communication between the call maker and the call receiver needs to be clear, concise and relevant (Higgins et al., 2001).

If you are in a position of working for NHS 111 or are undertaking telephone triage, it is important to note that some of the communication problems are associated with the emotional or physical state of the caller. The caller may be panicking, talk too quickly or be breathless, or they may not understand medical terms and jargon.

Delivering telehealth clearly requires specialist communication training, as well as an ability to stay calm under pressure and to be able to deal with callers who may be angry or upset. You would also need to work well with a team to communicate the callers' needs as clearly and concisely as possible. In Activity 4.3, there is an opportunity to think about what the key elements of communication via a telehealth platform are.

Activity 4.3   Communication: telehealth

You are working in the NHS 111 service and are a second line contact for the callers after the initial triage has been done by one of the administrative team members. The admin team member passes a call through to you with the following notes:

Date and time of call: 13/03/2022 17:45 Team member: Becky Cattaway

> Situation: Pts name is Tony not sure of gender. D.O.B 20 April 1969
>
> Address: 6 Springfield Road, Newton-on-Avon, NT66 6TX
>
> Tel: 0777789890
>
> Background: History of cough for the last four days, and some shortness of breath on exertion.
>
> Past medical history of asthma as a child. No recent surgery, no pain or swelling in either leg.
>
> Assessment: Temp, feel hot (has hot eyes), but does not have a thermometer. Cough is dry. Has taken paracetamol 20 minutes ago, does not feel better.
>
> Recommendations: Referral to qualified nursing staff made 17:54.

As the nurse receiving the call, what do you think you need to do or be aware of in general when communicating with a patient over the phone?

Suggested answers can be found at the end of this chapter.

Activity 4.3 looked at the challenges of remote communication and establishing a therapeutic relationship to provide care. We will move on now to the communication within the patient's home environment or accommodation.

At home

It is interesting to understand what 'home' means. It can be the place where your family reside or where you are most happy. It can also be where you permanently live. If we use the last definition of a home, we can apply this to many different care settings that would not be seen as a conventional home on a street behind a single front door. A home could be a home away from home and be temporary accommodation like a holiday caravan or a respite centre. If you are nursing in a coastal community with holidaymakers, you could be providing care in these temporary homes. You may also be faced with multi-occupancy homes and the challenges of confidentiality and a safe space to practise in these environments.

In terms of institution theory, the same issues apply, as in a general workplace, but those environmental rules will be personal to the patient whose home you are visiting. They will be subtle and more difficult to predict.

District nurses and Community Psychiatric Nurses (CPN)

Each home comes with its own unique set of hazards and risks. As a community nurse entering the patient's home, you must be vigilant, as well as professional and polite; you are a guest, after all. When a person is receiving care in their own home, this can create a vulnerable situation for them, as the patient's home becomes the nurse's workplace and the roles that each would traditionally hold are blurred. The nurse, who would usually be associated with a hospital or clinic, is suddenly in the person's home; this can influence the behaviour and decision-making process of the patient (Höglander et al., 2020)

Prison and detention centres

Being in prison or a detention centre cannot be considered a home in the true sense but, rather, a place a person is forced to reside. This environment is run by an authority who controls the will of the detainees. The rules and routines are strict and rigorously monitored and enforced. The norms are to conform with little free movement or free will.

People in prison have the same rights to healthcare as everyone else. The right to health is a fundamental human right and is protected within the European Convention on Human Rights, under Article 2 (right to life) and Article 3 (freedom from torture and inhuman or degrading treatment). Most prisons are set up to deal with most medical cases and may even have a few hospital beds in a specific medical area. These medical areas and services are staffed by doctors and nurses/nursing associates who will have experience in general medicine, as well as mental health and addiction care.

When reviewing government data on the prison system, there were 79,235 people living in one of the 121 prisons within the UK in 2020 (UK Prison Population Statistics, 2020). People who end up in prison may not have seen a GP for some time and may have untreated physical ailments. In addition, the Institute of Psychiatry estimates that over half of the prison population experience poor mental health and around 15% of these have the need for specialist mental health needs. It is thought that 2% have serious or acute mental health needs. In addition, the *Prison Drugs Strategy* published by HM Prison and Probation Service (2019) noted that, since 2017/2018, the positive results of random drug tests detecting a substance has increased by 50%.

If we consider for a moment the feelings you expressed from Activity 4.1 and the anxiousness associated with being admitted as an inpatient in a general hospital, apply this to being in prison. When you consider that a prison inmate is not permitted to wear their own clothes and has a strictly timed routine beyond their control with no means of freedom of movement, combined with loud noises and unfamiliar sounds, it is not hard to imagine the stress and terror which they may feel in this environment, particularly when all familiar personal contacts have been severed.

As a nursing professional within this environment, you will be required to have strong interpersonal skills, assertiveness, self-confidence, emotional intelligence and personal integrity and resilience. It is essential that you communicate in a confident manner but remain approachable and professional, with the ability to be assertive if needed. Saying no, or challenging unacceptable behaviour, can feel scary at first, but you will gain respect from both prisoners and staff. In Activity 4.4, you can explore the challenge of nursing in a secure environment.

Activity 4.4   Decision making

You are the nursing associate on duty in a category A prison and you receive an urgent message via the radio system to attend a cell on the third floor, which is two floors away from the medical centre.

What issues will you need to consider before you leave the medical centre to attend?

You arrive at the cell to find Greg, the individual you have been called to see, on the floor, clutching his stomach and complaining of pain. He is a 28-year-old man and has been in the prison for the last six months. You had seen him a few times for depression and anxiety prior to this.

Is there anything else you need to know at this point?

A security officer tells you that Greg has taken a large quantity of illicit drugs and that they needed access to the cell for a search. Greg confirms what the officer said about the drugs, but he is refusing help and states he wants to die.

What is your next step here?

You review Greg's physical observations, and you find that he has tachycardia (120 bpm), a raised temperature (38°C) and a fast respiratory rate (32 bpm). You also note he has a distended abdomen. It is clear that Greg is deteriorating and needs to get to hospital.

The security staffs tell you that they cannot escort him at this time because they were carrying out searches of the wing and the prison was on lockdown because they were concerned he was a security risk.

What are your next steps here?

Suggested answers can be found at the end of this chapter.

Activity 4.4 offered insight into working and providing care in a restrictive environment. As this chapter moves on, we will explore less restrictive options for care in different accommodation settings.

Supported living

Supported living offers an alternative to assisted living and residential care. It refers to a range of services and community living environments designed for individuals with conditions such as learning difficulties, autism, brain injuries or other complex care needs. This also extends to families with a disabled family member to support. The aim for those in a supported living setting is for them to retain their citizenship and independence and to be part of a community with assistance that is tailored to their needs.

There are four tiers of supported living:

Independent living

This is where someone can choose to live independently in their own flat with as much or as little support as needed.

Shared living

This is for those who want to live independently but aren't yet ready to live alone. They benefit from having their own space but also being able to socialise too. They share communal spaces and the cost of household bills.

Apartment living

This is for those who want to live independently in an apartment with some shared communal space, if they want to socialise. (See also the section on community-assisted living.)

Stepping-stone accommodation

This provides stability for those who are between long-term care environments. This type of accommodation gives the most support and helps the person to plan for their future in a structured way. The person is supported in developing the skills they may need to help them live more independently until they are ready to move onto the next stage.

In Activity 4.5, there is an opportunity to think about what tier of supported living would be appropriate for a new service user, and what questions you would need to ask in order to make a judgement on the level of support required.

Activity 4.5   Work-based learning and decision making

You are working in a large complex for clients with learning disabilities. The complex has a wide range of options for living environments and varying levels of support available.

Natasha Thomas is 55 years old and has been diagnosed with Prader-Willi syndrome. She has been institutionalised for 44 years in a variety of large district hospitals since she was 11 years old. Her current accommodation is closing down and the local Clinical Commissioning Group (CCG) plan for Natasha to have support in a community-based accommodation setting.

(Continued)

(Continued)

Spending a long time in an institution with structured routines and regimented rules will have impacted Natasha's ability and suitability for a community placement. You are having your first meeting with Natasha, and she is clearly anxious and appears angry. How would you approach Natasha here? For more information on Prader-Willi, refer to the useful websites section at the end of this chapter. Using a rationale for your choices, consider what questions you would need to ask to establish what level of support Natasha would need.

Suggested answers can be found at the end of the chapter.

In Activity 4.5, it is clear that there is a variation in needs relative to the services provided. How you can adequately support people who are transitioning from one care environment to another requires an in-depth assessment.

Community-assisted living

Community-based homes vary vastly from an assisted living environment where the residents have a high degree of autonomy, in comparison to a nursing home where a resident's complex needs require nursing interventions and the resident is dependent.

Assisted living is for older people or people with disabilities who can live fairly independently, but who need some help with everyday tasks and some means of additional support from a warden or support team.

The common features of assisted living accommodation include:

- a 24-hour emergency call system;
- self-contained flats within a bigger complex;
- communal areas to socialise;
- some social activities.

The nursing associate's role in this setting is as a supporter and facilitator, and communication skills are essential to that role. Please also see the section on district nurses and Community Psychiatric Nurses (CPN) on p. 67.

Care home or nursing home

Good communication makes residents feel cared for; it puts them at ease and promotes dignity (Social Care Institute for Excellence (SCIE), 2020). A residential or nursing home poses challenges for communication because it is not only the resident's home but also a working environment.

Effective communication in this environment not only improves care delivery but also creates a better working culture by encouraging openness and transparency. Because of this, it makes both the healthcare team feel more empowered and motivated, and the care is better coordinated.

Within this environment, you must recognise that the residents will require support and clear communication to support them in their transition from a state of total independence to being a member of a multiple occupancy site. Assisting someone to adapt their lifestyle requires understanding and patience.

Community homes like hospital wards are busy and noisy places. Noisy activities, from the cleaner vacuuming the hall carpet to a squeaky wheel on the tea trolley, all impact on communication. As we have seen in Chapter 1, there are interruptions to combat too, from other residents wanting your attention to other staff in need of your assistance. You need to be aware of these barriers and distractions to effective communication and should be able to take simple steps to limit any interference. In Activity 4.6, we will look at how to manage some simple distractions in a care home setting.

Activity 4.6   Communication

Mrs Kelly is a new resident in the 28-bedded mixed nursing and care home. There are ten nursing home beds and 18 care home beds. Mrs Kelly is in room 12, which is a front-facing double occupancy room on the first floor, which she shares with Mrs Eveleigh.

Mrs Kelly is upset and is finding it hard to adapt to this new environment in a busy town, away from her rural bungalow, which she has just heard has been sold. Mrs Kelly and Mrs Eveleigh get on well enough, but Mrs Kelly is struggling to cope with how loud Mrs Eveleigh has the television, due to Mrs Eveleigh's deafness.

You are the nursing associate in charge of the first floor and you are going to talk to Mrs Kelly. What steps are you going to take in managing the physical environment so that you can optimise your communication with Mrs Kelly?

Answers to this activity can be found at the end of the chapter.

Activity 4.6 has explored the impact of the physical environment and some simple measures you can do to enhance communication. Environmental control is very important for residents experiencing fluctuating mental capacity, confusion or living with dementia. You should:

- remove all distractions if possible, such as turning off the television or radio;
- find a quiet space where the person can focus more;
- engage with family members and loved ones on how they communicate with the person. Make this a care plan action and record steps needed.

Chapter 7 will explore the impact of cognitive problems, such as dementia, how it can affect care decisions and what you as a nursing associate can do to protect the patient.

Chapter summary

In this chapter, we have explored some of the areas in which nursing and care delivery takes place most commonly. We have looked at some of the issues relevant to those environments and communication. There will be regional variations to communication for you to consider that are specific to your working area and setting. It is useful that you reflect on the activities within this chapter and try and put yourself in the position of the patient/service user in those different settings to help you experience their perceptions and understand their anxieties.

Activities: Brief outline answers

Activity 4.2 Work-based learning (page 65)

In the first instance, Archie's grandfather cannot give permission for the immunisations to take place if he does not have the permission of the legal guardian or is not the legal guardian of the child himself. It would be good practice to check whether the grandfather has a letter from Archie's mother stating that she is happy for the vaccinations to take place. It needs to be dated and signed.

In the absence of a letter, it would be worth checking to see if Archie's mother was in the waiting room and able and willing to join you in the clinic room to give parental consent for the immunisations to go ahead.

If there is no letter, she refuses to join you in the clinic or is absent, the appointment will need to be concluded without giving Archie his vaccinations. You would need to make sure that the appointment is re-booked within the next few days and that the grandfather is fully aware of what needs to happen for next time.

It might also be worth getting the family to read some information on vaccinations in the time between the next appointment. A valuable source is the NHS vaccinations webpage: **www.nhs.uk/conditions/vaccinations/6-in-1-infant-vaccine/**

It could be a good idea to make sure the next appointment is a little longer, so you have time to discuss the difference in the polio vaccine as an injection rather than the oral application. It would also allow for the asking of questions.

Activity 4.3 Communication: telehealth (page 66)

- Prepare for the call: get your information ready. Look for pages on asthma, Covid-19 symptoms and chest infections.
- Make sure you are talking to the right person: confidentiality matters.
- Ask how they would like to be addressed/what you should call them.
- Make sure you have a contact telephone number, so if you get disconnected, you can call them back. Check the number on file with the caller.
- Be clear about the purpose of the call: what is the aim of the call?

- Remember there are no non-verbal cues they can pick up on: they cannot see you either.
- Check your tone of voice: this may differ depending on the nature of the call.
- Listen carefully: you could take notes.
- Speak clearly and succinctly: get to the point without being blunt.
- If you didn't hear what they said, or you don't understand, ask for clarity.
- Summarise the conversation and make your recommendations known to the caller: ask them if they agree with the summary and check that they have understood it.
- Ask them whether there is anything else you can do for them.

Activity 4.4 Decision-making (page 68)

What issues will you need to consider before you leave the medical centre to attend?

- The equipment you need to take with you.
- How long it is going to take to get there (through many locked gates) and the quickest route.
- Logging off the computer.
- Locking the medical centre office.
- Whether it is safe to attend.
- Whether you are leaving someone at risk alone.
- Whether you are the best person to attend.

Is there anything else you need to know when you arrive at the cell?

- Is it safe to enter the cell?
- Will a security team member be attending with you?

What is your next step when Greg states that he wants to die?

- Establish capacity.
- Does he know what he has taken?
- How long ago was it taken?
- Conduct a full A–E assessment, if he consents.

What are your next steps when you realise Greg needs to get to the hospital but the security staff say they cannot escort him?

- Communicate with Greg your findings and the plan.
- Continue to advocate for the patient.
- Maintain the patient's safety.
- Escalate the request for hospital transfer through the management structure.

Activity 4.5 Work-based learning and decision making (page 69)

Temper outbursts are common for people with Prader-Willi, particularly when they are under stress or are experiencing a change in routine or plan.

A technique to use here is to 'switch' Natasha's focus from the change in routine to something else and ideally more pleasurable. It is important Natasha knows you are not disappointed or upset with her, as she is likely to feel upset about the outburst later.

Using pictures, images and objects can help focus Natasha onto another topic, which should break the cycle of the outburst.

Using a rationale for your choices, consider what questions you would need to ask to establish what level of support Natasha would need.

- Natasha is going to need a structure that is not too removed from what she is currently used to, but one that can be adjusted in time, if needed. So, you will need to ask questions about what that routine is.
- She should be asked about her choices, but be mindful that she may not know what choices are available to her. It is most likely she will want to stick to the familiar because change can be difficult, but not impossible with the right support. You will need to ask what she is used to doing.
- Certain aspects such as shopping, preparing food, cooking, doing laundry, doing housework, and managing her finances or managing her own medications, are all going to be new concepts for Natasha. Also, considering the young age that she was institutionalised, it may be that she has never been shopping or does not have much of a concept of money. You will need to ask questions to establish her understanding of these aspects.
- You are also going to need to consider her safety. If she is suddenly in an environment where she is free to move around and access the outside, will she wander and does she have the ability for self-preservation?
- Is she able to self-care and manage her own hygiene?
- Communication needs. Can she read and write?
- What are Natasha's interests/hobbies/recreational/social activities/religious/ spiritual needs?

This is not an exhaustive list.

Activity 4.6 Communication (page 71)

In the first instance, you may need to delegate your current task to a suitably competent and qualified person.

Communicate with your team and tell them where you will be and what you will be doing. Ask them not to disturb you unless it is important.

Communicate to the team the person you have allocated as an alternative contact who will be referred to for questions/help/support in your absence, while talking to Mrs Kelly.

Go to room 12 and knock on the door and ask if it is okay to enter.

The next step is to ensure privacy. If Mrs Eveleigh is willing and able, you could politely ask her to leave for a few minutes; she would not be obligated to do so as this is her room and her home just as much as it is Mrs Kelly's.

If Mrs Eveleigh is happy to give you a few minutes, thank her for her consideration.

If Mrs Eveleigh is not prepared to leave the room, it is important you find somewhere else for you and Mrs Kelly to talk.

Turn the television/radio off or down enough for it not to be a distraction.

Is there external noise? It may be necessary to close the window and close the door from noises outside of the room.

Knowledge review

Now that you have worked through the chapter, how would you rate your knowledge of the following topics?

	Good	Adequate	Poor
• the four fields of nursing			
• some of the settings where nursing takes place			
• some of the factors that help achieve effective communication			
• barriers to communication by setting			
• whom institutional theory can impact on communication			

If you are unsure of some aspects, what are you going to do next?

Further reading and useful websites

You can find more information on life in prison at the following government links:
www.gov.uk/life-in-prison
https://data.justice.gov.uk/prisons

For information on the pressures on general practice:
**www.bma.org.uk/advice-and-support/nhs-delivery-and-workforce/
pressures/pressures-in-general-practice**
**www.rcgp.org.uk/-/media/Files/News/2019/RCGP-fit-for-the-future-report-
may-2019.ashx?la=en**

For information on the experiences of adult inpatients:
www.cqc.org.uk/publications/surveys/adult-inpatient-survey-2019

For further information on who can give consent:
https://assets.publishing.service.gov.uk/government/uploads/system/uploads/attachment_data/file/144250/Green-Book-Chapter-2-Consent-PDF-77K.pdf

For further information on staff debriefing:
www.talkdebrief.org/talkhome

For more information on Prader-Willi syndrome:
www.findresources.co.uk/the-syndromes/prader-willi/key-facts

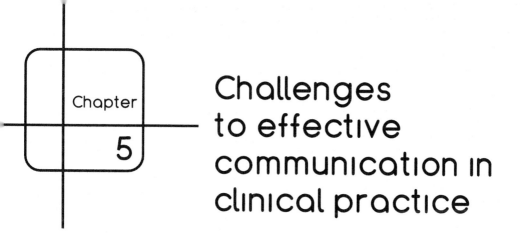

Challenges to effective communication in clinical practice

NMC FUTURE NURSE STANDARDS OF PROFICIENCY FOR NURSING ASSOCIATES

This chapter will address the following platforms and proficiencies:

Platform 1: Being an accountable professional

At the point of registration, the nursing associate will be able to:

1.5 understand the demands of professional practice and demonstrate how to recognise signs of vulnerability in themselves or their colleagues and the action required to minimise risks to health.

1.10 demonstrate the skills and abilities required to develop, manage and maintain appropriate relationships with people, their families, carers and colleagues.

Platform 3: Provide and monitor care

At the point of registration, the nursing associate will be able to:

3.7 demonstrate and apply an understanding of how and when to escalate to the appropriate professional for expert help and advice.

3.8 demonstrate and apply an understanding of how people's needs for safety, dignity, privacy, comfort and sleep can be met.

3.13 demonstrate an understanding of how to deliver sensitive and compassionate end-of-life care to support people to plan for their end of life, giving information and support to people who are dying, their families and the bereaved. Provide care to the deceased.

Annexe A: Communication and relationship management skills

At the point of registration, the nursing associate will be able to safely demonstrate the following skills:

(Continued)

(Continued)

2. Communication skills for supporting people to prevent ill health and manage their health challenges:

2.9 engage in difficult conversations with support from others, helping people who are feeling emotionally or physically vulnerable or in distress, conveying compassion and sensitivity.

Chapter aims

By the end of this chapter, you will be able to:

- understand the challenge of communication with people in heightened emotional states.
- consider how to de-escalate an angry communication.
- consider how to approach difficult conversations.
- explore empathic communication.
- define and explore the causes of aggression and violence.

Introduction

Communication in many instances can become defensive and lead to destructive behaviours and broken relationships. Learning how to predict and prevent an escalation to violence supports the patient and protects your team. Communication is a fundamental feature of successful nursing, which cannot be taken for granted. Although communication is a skill, it is a skill that is never mastered and is only ever improved upon. As you engage with colleagues and service users, the uniqueness of those communications enhances your skills and informs your understanding of the needs of people and awareness of the barriers to communication. Within this chapter, you will be exploring the skills required to successfully communicate with persons in a heightened state of emotion and upset. You will start with understanding aggression and violence and how it may be prevented, as well as how you can calm and de-escalate a situation. Particular reference is made to managing a person experiencing a manic mental state, moving on finally to the exploration of death, dying and expressions of grief.

Healthcare encounters are often emotionally charged events which can be either positive or negative. Positive encounters, from a pregnancy announcement for a couple who have had trouble conceiving, to an all-clear on the test results after cancer treatment, are those we take delight in and look forward to. Negative encounters, however, are more common and can be related to fear, worry, pain and distress (Ali, 2017). You can explore other aspects that may influence your behaviour in Activity 5.1.

Activity 5.1   Critical thinking

Take ten minutes to think about what aspects of life have shaped the way you behave. You might want to think about your family and your life growing up. Who has influenced you the most and how?

An outline answer is provided at the end of the chapter, although this remains subjective and personal to your experiences.

Distress and upset

Aggression

You have seen in Activity 5.1 that there are many different influences on your behaviour, some of which may have shaped what makes you upset or angry. A firm definition of aggression is harder to establish because aggression can take many forms and have many reasons, but the expression of aggression usually consists of one or more of the following elements:

- an expression of energy;
- a display of immoral, repulsive or inappropriate behaviour;
- an intention to cause harm, to damage or hurt someone physically or psychologically;
- the intention to dominate someone or others;
- an expression of anger;
- defensive or protective behaviour;
- verbal abuse, derogatory talk, threats or non-verbal gestures;
- a threat to acquire something or reach a goal;
- the damaging of objects or the environment, from vandalism to smashing plates and crockery;
- a means to physically injure or kill someone with or without the use of weapons;
- forcing someone to do something against their will;
- an inappropriate, unwanted or rejected sexual display or contact.

(National Institute of Clinical Excellence (NICE) 2015).

You can see from the list that aggressive behaviour is broadly intended to cause physical or emotional harm to either person(s) or property. Similarly, with the many different motivations for aggression, there are different types of aggression. There is dispute in the academic world about whether there are only two types of aggression or whether there are three types, and a recent definition could be considered and included in the debate. In this section, you will have an opportunity to review all the main theories around types of aggression which have been subject to research.

We start with social psychologists who look at how the thoughts, feelings and behaviours of individuals are influenced by the presence of others, whether real or imagined. They have concluded that there are only two types of aggression (Bushman and Anderson, 2001). These are:

Emotional or impulsive aggression

This is aggression that happens suddenly and unpredictably, with very little time to think about it, and is often associated with negative emotions. An example of impulsive aggression can be seen in road rage. This is defined as aggressive or angry behaviour exhibited by motorists. These behaviours often include verbal insults, physical threats or dangerous driving that is targeted towards either another driver or non-drivers, such as pedestrians or cyclists. It is an explosive emotion intended to release frustration immediately.

Instrumental or cognitive aggression

In opposition to emotional aggression, instrumental or cognitive aggression is planned and intentional. It is often associated with an aim to hurt someone to gain something. A terrorist who plans, makes and plants a bomb intended to kill civilians in order to draw attention to a political cause would be an example of instrumental or cognitive aggression (Bushman and Anderson, 2001).

On the other hand, psychologists who study normal and abnormal mental states have generally accepted there to be three types of aggression. These are:

Reactive-expressive

Like emotional or impulsive aggression, reactive-expressive aggression behaviour is unplanned, impulsive and usually a response to a direct or perceived threat. This can be displayed as verbal or physical aggression or a combination of the two, and it is directed at the source of the threat.

Reactive-inexpressive

This is a defensive form of aggression which forms the basis of hostility or passive aggressive behaviours. The emotional anger which drives this form of aggression is suppressed and released indirectly, such as by avoiding direct or clear communication, making excuses, blaming others, being obstructive, playing the victim, sarcasm or backhanded compliments.

Proactive-relational

Proactive-relational aggression, another covert or suppressed form of aggression, seeks to harm a person by damaging their reputation or manipulating their relationships. This type of behaviour is planned and goal orientated, like instrumental or cognitive aggression. However, this form of aggression is intended to break human relationships, for example, by spreading nasty rumours (Kawabata et al., 2016).

Lastly, following the increasing rates of school bullying, the most recent form of aggression is recognised by some to be cyberbullying. This aggression is displayed through the use of computers, mobile phones and other electronic devices (Hinduja and Patchin, 2009).

It is clear that whatever type of aggression a person is displaying, aggressive behaviour damages social boundaries. It can lead to breakdowns in relationships, and it can be obvious or secretive. Occasional aggressive outbursts are common and even normal in the right circumstances. As a nursing associate, you have to be able to identify and understand the causes of aggressive behaviour so you can have awareness of when violence might occur. You will also need to consider that certain conditions can contribute to aggressive behaviour. An expression of aggression is not solely due to an emotional display but can have a clinical cause. In Activity 5.2, you can start thinking about some of those clinical causes of aggression.

Activity 5.2   Critical thinking

Different health conditions can contribute to aggression behaviour. What disorders or conditions can you think of that might have a contributing factor in a display of aggression?

An outline answer is provided at the end of the chapter.

Following Activity 5.2, you will have seen that there is a wide range of clinical conditions that can prompt an aggressive display. Relative to communication and care delivery, it is important to understand that aggression, when not checked or challenged, can escalate to violence.

Violence

Understanding the impact that violence has in healthcare is important to establish how communication is critical to its resolution. Violence is defined by the World Health Organisation in the *World Report on Violence and Health* (Krug et al., 2002) as 'the intentional use of physical force or power, threatened or actual, against oneself, another person, or against a group or community, that either results in or has a high likelihood of resulting in injury, death, psychological harm, maldevelopment or deprivation.'

The Health and Safety Executive (HSE) defines work-related violence as 'any incident in which a person is abused, threatened or assaulted in circumstances relating to their work' (1996). Verbal abuse and threats are the most common types of incident. Physical attacks are comparatively rare.

When you think of violence in the NHS, you would likely think of the paramedics on a Friday or Saturday night, when the drunk young men and women on an evening out clash, then the staff in A&E when those patched-up revellers spill out of the ambulances and into the department. This is a stereotypical assumption based on tabloid media coverage and fly-on-the-wall sensationalised television programming.

In fact, mental health nurses are more at risk, and most violent incidents occur between 10:00 and 11:00 (Department of Health and Social Care, 2018). However, the demographic most likely to be involved in violent and aggressive incidents is men aged between 75–95 (Harwood, 2017).

Environment

Preventing difficulties

Research has shown that good communication can have a beneficial impact in challenging environments where aggression and violence can be triggered (Neades, 2013). Keeping waiting patients informed of the expected time before they are seen can set an initial expectation, but failure to communicate an extension to that waiting time will cause upset and unrest if the initial time is exceeded.

Acknowledging the waiting time with a simple statement such as 'I am sorry you have had to wait so long' and keeping information channels friendly and open can prevent an escalation.

In longer-stay care environments, try to make a connection by identifying common ground with your patients. Acknowledging them as an individual (National Institute for Health and Care Excellence, 2021) helps the patients understand you are an individual too. Using observational and listening skills, along with friendly, reassuring chats, can help identify situations that may escalate and become aggressive (Ali, 2018). Activity 5.3 asks you to think about how a person might be communicating to you that they are angry.

Activity 5.3   Case study

Angela is 27 years old and is living in a multi-occupancy community residential home for individuals with a range of learning difficulties. She is well liked and can live fairly independently, with some assistance and support from the community home team.

Angela's father has just arrived at the home to drop Angela off, after she had spent the weekend with her family. After slamming the car door, Angela walks past you without speaking and enters the home. Following behind her, you notice that she has left her bags in the hallway. A few minutes later, you hear shouting from the communal area. You enter and see Angela pacing the room with her arms folded. One of the other residents complains to you that Angela swore at her and kicked the chair they were sitting in. Angela rushes over, points her finger into the other resident's face and calls them a liar. You tell Angela to step back and ask the other resident if they are okay. Angela is heard to copy your words using a childlike tone to mimic you.

Which of Angela's behaviours makes you think she is communicating anger or upset?

An outline answer is provided at the end of the chapter.

Having recognised some of the signs that someone is getting agitated and angry from Activity 5.3, you need to consider what you are now going to do about it. This section will explore the most common and consistent aspects of several de-escalation techniques.

De-escalation

You have already seen, in this chapter, that there are many conditions and situations that can be a contributing factor in aggression and violence. You also know that health settings are prone to frequent feelings of upset, anxiety and aggression that can lead to violence if unchallenged or if communication is inadequate.

Approach

You have seen, throughout the book, that communication is central to relationships and making connections with people. So, before you approach the person who is displaying signs of anger, it is important that you establish that it is safe to proceed towards them in order to form a connection as soon as possible. You will do this by introducing yourself and by using their name regularly during the communication. Your aim, in the first instance, is just to try and calm the situation down by using a gentle, calm tone of voice, and slower movements and gestures reduce the tension in the communication. Treat the person with dignity and respect, even if this is not being given to you; ignore insults and do not be judgemental.

When you have their attention, you can ask questions, asking only one question at a time and giving them ample time to answer you before moving on. The questions themselves should be worded so as not to devalue or invalidate their feelings. So, instead of 'I can't see why you are angry' or 'how are you feeling?' – because that will be obvious and both questions are likely to inflame the situation – it is better to say, for example, 'I notice you are angry' (Lowry and Lingard, 2016).

You may also consider using an open question such as, 'Help me to understand what you are upset about.' This makes the person think about the cause of the problem, which will offer you options towards a solution.

Body language

Referring back to Chapter 1, when you read about body language, we can apply what was learned there in the context of communication during de-escalation. While maintaining a calm demeanour, and with an open posture, face the person, making sure you are allowing space between you and them. Wherever possible, position yourself at the same level as the person, so that eye contact is easy. Do be aware, however, to consider what the appropriate level of eye contact to use is. While it is important to establish eye contact, constant staring should be avoided. Equally the use of smiling should be considered carefully. Smile if it is appropriate; if not, maintain a neutral expression.

To maintain a non-threatening posture, incline your head slightly and nod occasionally. A nod demonstrates your attention and your willingness to listen without interrupting.

Assess risk

From earlier in this chapter, you have some context of how aggression can escalate to violence, as well as the costs that has on the individuals involved and the healthcare service. Having awareness of the potential risks in a situation and the background of the person, if known, is valuable knowledge when needing to attempt communication.

The paramount concern in situations that have the potential to break down is the safety of all the participants and whether the person is a risk to themselves or others. You should consider whether you need assistance and how you are going to summon assistance. Being conscious of your surroundings, think about whether you can leave the room safely. Is the person experiencing the distress safe; if not, can you move them to a place of safety?

It may be that, if a situation is volatile to the extent that initial communication has little effect, it is necessary to either offer tranquilisers, perform rapid tranquilisation or use a restrictive practice or restraint as a last resort.

Environment

Similar to assessing risk, the continued awareness of the environment and the space you are in is important. As discussed in Chapter 3, we should be looking to minimise distractions by turning off the television and reducing noises. Wherever possible, take them to a quiet space, invite them to sit down and ensure you respect their privacy and dignity at all times.

Understanding and empathy

When someone is expressing hostility towards you, it is difficult to maintain composure and remain empathetic and understanding. As a professional nursing associate, you are required to:

1.10 demonstrate the skills and abilities required to develop, manage and maintain appropriate relationships with people, their families, carers and colleagues.

3.4 demonstrate the knowledge, communication and relationship management skills required to provide people, families and carers with accurate information that meets their needs before, during and after a range of interventions.

When someone is showing signs of hostility, as you have seen in Activity 5.3, it is important you maintain effective communication and prevent an escalation. Can you think about a time when you have been angry and the person talking to you keeps interrupting you and finishing your sentences for you? I am sure you can reflect on feeling irritated by the interruptions and how they stopped you from making your feelings heard. Those same feelings apply to patients you are communicating with, and their significant others, if they are upset or angry.

Having the ability to reflect on your own communications can give you insight into how best to communicate. If you feel uncomfortable with a communication, a good technique is to count slowly down from ten in your head. This should give you enough time to regain some composure and give you space to think of your next move.

Leaving space in a communication by counting down from ten in your head is also a good mechanism to encourage the other person to speak. As we saw in Chapter 3, there is power in silence. Try to avoid the temptation to fill those silences between you with words.

When the person does communicate with you, it is important you make sure they feel like they are being heard. An example of this can be seen in the next section and can be done by paraphrasing, which is the method of using different words to repeat what the person has just told you.

The following dialogue will be used as a basis for the following steps in communication and will be referred back to.

Patient: 'I have been waiting here for over an hour and a half for my appointment and no one is telling me anything. It is getting ridiculous, and I am in pain!'

Nursing associate (paraphrasing): 'So you have been waiting a long time for your appointment and you are uncomfortable and would like to know what is happening.'

When listening and making someone feel heard, you can also make brief comments on the concerns they express, but don't offer a solution, don't make promises, or provide an explanation.

Using the previous example, a comment you may choose to use is the following:

Nursing associate (brief comment): 'I can imagine you feel frustrated by the long wait.'

Once communication has been established, it is important you allow the patient to retain 'ownership' of the problem and give them choices as to how to move forward towards a solution.

Nursing associate (allowing the patient to retain ownership): 'I would like to help you; how can I help?'

Patient: 'I want you to find out how much longer I have to wait.'

The nursing associate in this example now has a task to perform. The important aspect here is to set some expectations on how long this task will take to perform, who needs to be involved in completing it and what potential barriers there are, and that essentially you will keep them informed of your progress by checking back in with them. Be mindful that patients are likely to get angry again within 90 minutes of the initial outburst (Murphy, 2001).

Using the example dialogue, we will set the expectations:

Nursing associate (setting expectations): 'I will need to speak to the doctor in the clinic, but I will have to wait until she has finished seeing the patient with her right now. Hopefully, that won't take too long, and I should be able to get into the clinic room within the next ten minutes. If there is any delay, I will let you know.'

The example dialogue we have focused on in this section is a common interaction that should be easily resolved without escalation. We should acknowledge that good relationships can emerge from difficult beginnings. Patients often feel more appreciative towards a nurse when they have shared an experience that has had a satisfactory resolution (Price et al., 2015).

Having looked at what skills are required in preventing an escalation, you will have an opportunity in Activity 5.4 to explore a scenario and think about how you would manage the communication and others involved.

Activity 5.4   Interprofessional team working

You are the registered nursing associate on an early shift with a team of assorted healthcare professionals. You are working on an 18-bedded mixed-sex inpatient ward, specialising in care of the elderly with dementia.

It is 10:15. You hear slightly raised voices and you think someone is crying in one of the four bed bays near the end of the corridor.

The phone rings and you answer it. It is the bed manager, who wants to know your availability. During the call, the voices get louder, and you are certain now someone is crying. You do not end the call but delegate the task of investigating the noises to a healthcare support worker (HCSW).

A few moments later, you hear a scream from the same direction as the previous voices.

1. What are your next steps?

The raised voices continue, so you investigate. On entering the bay, you see a male patient standing near the end of the bed of a female patient with the HCSW between the two. The female patient is sitting in her bedside chair, cowering and crying. The male patient is stood with a walking stick in his hand, swinging it about above his head. He is repeatedly shouting for the female patient to 'Shut up!'

The HCSW is standing with her hands on her hips, facing the male patient, and she is loudly telling the patient to 'Go and sit down! Now!' The female patient screams as the male patient lunges towards her. The HCSW pushes the male patient back and away, and in that moment, he hits her with the walking stick across the shoulder.

2. What are your next steps and what is your priority?

With the assistance of the registered nurse, you get the male patient back to his bay and sitting in his bedside chair. As he sees the familiar bedside objects, he starts to calm down and becomes tearful and upset.

3. What are your next steps?

After a few minutes of sitting with the male patient without speaking and just listening to what he is saying, it is clear that he had walked into the wrong bay after using the bathroom. He thought that the female patient was in his bed, and he wanted her to move.

4. What would you say?

The male patient is now calm. The female patient is uninjured and is also now calm, following the registered nurse's support. Both patients have their call bells close to hand and are safe.

5. What should happen now and what are you going to focus on?

An outline answer is provided at the end of the chapter.

In Activity 5.4, you looked at managing an aggressive outburst and de-escalation. You will now explore the opposite end of the spectrum and the management of patients with mania.

Mental health conditions with mania

It is estimated that between one and five people will experience at least one episode of mania and 1% of them will need admission to hospital. Most people who experience mania have bipolar disorder, which could manifest as a mild depression only (NHS Choices, 2019).

Mania has been defined by WHO (1992) into three different degrees. They are each characterised by certain behaviours. Hypomania is the mildest form of mania, where the patient is not unwell enough to be admitted to hospital. Next, there is mania without psychosis, where the patient may require hospitalisation, but does not display psychotic symptoms such as delusion or hallucinations. Mania without psychosis is also referred to as bipolar I, which is a disorder where a person has had at least one manic episode in their life. A manic episode is a period of abnormally elevated high energy or irritability that is found in conjunction with other abnormal behaviours that disrupt life.

There may also be secondary causes, such as substance abuse, which can be a cause of mania without psychosis, and which would not be diagnosed as a bipolar I disorder.

Lastly, there is mania with psychosis. This can be mistaken for schizophrenia as the person experiences hallucinations and delusions. This is a bipolar II disorder that involves a serious depressive episode lasting for at least two weeks with at least one hypomanic episode. Hypomania is characterised by notable behaviour changes that are significantly different from the person's typical or normal behaviour.

Hypomania is commonly displayed as unusual excitement, flamboyance, irritability or aggression, along with feelings of restlessness and extreme talkativeness. It can also be associated with a reduced inhibition, inappropriate sexual behaviour and increased risk-taking activities, like excessive spending and grandiose ideas (Thomas and Mathias, 2000, cited in McColm et al., 2006).

With communication in mind, the challenges come when trying to convince someone who is feeling or experiencing something truly amazing and exciting that they are in fact quite unwell and are living with a mental health disorder.

If the person is considered a risk to themselves or others, or if they are at risk from others while they are in this vulnerable state (McColm et al., 2006), it may be necessary in the first instance to take initial action and detain them in hospital under section 2 of the Mental Health Act (HMSO, 1983). It may also be necessary to engage in rapid tranquilisation. It is good practice to check your employers' policies on such events before they happen.

The maintenance of the therapeutic relationship with the person experiencing a manic episode is difficult and does require frequent staff changes and self-awareness to counter the effects of the 'intoxicating exuberance' of the manic state. The interprofessional team should work together to ensure the safety of the patient and the wellbeing of the carer in such a situation.

In some instances, it is necessary to use restraint when communication attempts cannot resolve aggression. The use of restraint had been commonplace, whether that is physical restraint or a chemical one with the use of sedatives. Patient safety concerns following the use of restraint included death because of positional **asphyxia** and symptoms of post-traumatic stress on the person restrained (Price et al., 2015). This practice remains in use but is a last resort, subject to strict control, training and monitoring. The topic of the use of restraint is outside the remit of this book, but more information can be found in the further information and useful reading section of this chapter.

The serious consequences following restraint resulted in the prioritisation of non-physical approaches, and there are many methods of de-escalation available. De-escalation essentially means 'to bring down'. The rationale for de-escalation is to prevent aggressive and dangerous situations from occurring and, in some situations, reduce the need for restrictive intervention.

De-escalation should start when the first signs of agitation, irritation, anger or aggression are recognised (NICE, 2015).

After the initial crisis intervention, the treatment of someone experiencing a manic episode requires a patient-centred therapeutic relationship. As the period of mania subsides, it is good practice to involve patients in the debrief. This can be done separately to the staff debrief or can be part of a joint debrief. The intention of the patient debrief is to help them understand the insight into the episode. When the patient emerges from the manic episode, they are likely to feel ashamed and uncomfortable. Your presence as a constant empathic, respectful voice will aid their recovery, by grounding them to reality and the present.

The early identification of clear boundaries helps develop trust between the patient and the carer, and it requires close observation. Every effort should be made to reduce stimulation, but do allow for 10–15 minutes of calm exercise daily. Do not engage with or endorse the delusion and maintain an empathetic and respectful communication throughout (McColm et al., 2006).

As the chapter moves along, we shall focus on a different type of situation that can cause distress and upset, and this is in the management of communication when someone is experiencing a loss or the death of a loved one. In Activity 5.5, there is an opportunity to reflect on a loss or a death that you have experienced.

Activity 5.5   Reflection

Take ten minutes to think about a time when you have lost someone in your life. This could be from a death, but could also be from a breakdown in a relationship, for example.

How did you feel when the loss occurred? What emotions did you experience?

Also think about what you did to move past the initial feelings.

An outline answer is provided at the end of the chapter, although this remains subjective and personal to your experiences.

In Activity 5.5, there was an opportunity to reflect on your emotions during a time of loss. These feelings will be similar to those you are caring for as they die or their life changes and for those who are left by that loss or change. Having the ability to understand what a person may be feeling is the essence of compassion.

As part of the process of reflection, you may have thought about how you found out about the lost or of when you heard that your loved one had a life-limiting diagnosis. A nursing associate, as part of a wider team, will most likely be involved in breaking bad news and supporting people with coming to terms with that news.

Bad news is usually associated with the end of life; however, it is not restricted to it. Bad news can be any communication of information which challenges or changes the person's view of the future in a negative way (Rosenzweig, 2012). It is not surprising that the nature of breaking bad news is an emotionally charged event for both the communication sender and receiver, and many healthcare professionals do not feel adequately equipped with the communication skills required, they are often usure about the amount of 'truth' to disclose and are afraid of causing pain or negativity to the patient and their loved ones (Narayanan et al., 2010).

When discussing death, the healthcare professional can be reminded of their own mortality and feel powerless to help those in emotional distress with their words (Narayanan et al., 2010). Death and discussion surrounding death remains taboo and there is insufficient training to ensure healthcare professionals are skilful in breaking bad news. This was particularly relevant during the Covid-19 pandemic whereby people were unable to support their loved ones in hospital. Breaking bad news is increasingly done over the phone and in remote circumstances (Collini et al., 2021).

In acknowledgement of the need for supporting healthcare professionals in delivering bad news, several models of breaking bad news have been developed. The SPIKES protocol (Baile et al., 2000) is the most used model and is a structured listening model that focuses on what the patient wants to know. It allows for information to be given in manageable amounts, allows for reactions to the news, checks the patient's understanding and offers support.

The acronym SPIKES stands for Setting up, Perception, Invitation, Knowledge, Emotions with Empathy and Strategy or Summary.

1. Firstly, establish an appropriate setting.

Where possible, seek somewhere quiet where you will not be disturbed. Take the time to prepare yourself for the conversation so as not to appear nervous or anxious. Take some time to be aware of your body language and eye contact. Refer back to Chapter 1 for more information.

2. Check the patient's perception of the situation, prompting the news regarding the illness or test results. Use this as a gentle way to initiate a conversation.

Using statements like 'Unfortunately I have some bad news to tell you,' or 'I am sorry to tell you,' or 'Things are not going in the direction we had hoped,' allows the patient and latterly family to emotionally brace themselves for the information that is to follow.

(Rosenzweig, 2012)

3.   Determine the amount of information known or how much information is desired.

As we will see in the next section on death, in grief and dying, there are a range of emotions and psychological states that people go through when processing bad news. The skill here is to employ empathic communication skills in establishing what stage they are at, as this will have an impact on what a person is prepared listen to. As an example, the patient might be in a state of bargaining where every statement of medical fact will be countered by 'what if' questions.

Here, you can invite others into the discussion by asking permission to share the news with their support network.

4.   Know the medical facts and their implication before initiating the conversation.

Be prepared and know what the diagnosis and treatment/comfort options there are before you start. You don't want to give half of the information, leaving people anxious and upset, only to have to start another breaking bad news conversation.

5.   Explore the emotions raised during the interview and respond with empathy.

Understandably the patients will respond with a wide range of potential emotions, and you should demonstrate empathic communications skills by expressing understanding of those emotions and respecting the difficulty of the situation.

Aligned with being prepared, make sure you have some tissues stored discreetly, but within easy reach (just outside the door or curtain, for example).

6.   Establish a strategy for support.

Checking the patient's understanding of what they have been told is important here. Before planning on a treatment plan or the next steps, you need to be certain that the patient is prepared for such a discussion. It might be necessary to give them some time to process and think about what has been said; however, you do not want to leave the conversation with no end.

The conversation should conclude with a plan and some understanding of the next steps, even if that plan is to come back and talk to you again tomorrow morning (Baile et al., 2000, cited in Rosenzweig, 2012).

Once the bad news has been given, the person must process the thoughts and feelings surrounding that news and make a 'new' life or develop a new understanding of life. These stages are also not exclusive to a situation involving death. Any traumatic incident or life-changing event, such as the break-up of a marriage, the birth of a disabled child or caring for someone with deteriorating dementia, can be associated with a loss and can be grieved in the same way as a death.

Death, grief and dying

Elizabeth Kübler-Ross (1969) is the founder of research surrounding death and dying. From her book *On Death and Dying*, we learn that there are five stages to death, dying and grief (see Figure 5.1).

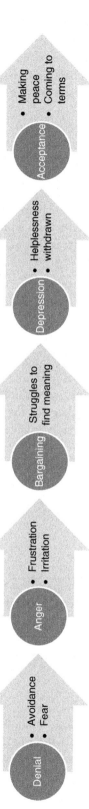

Figure 5.1 Stages of death and dying, the common feelings and the needs of the dying patient and their significant others.

It is important to note that not everyone will follow the linear example given here. Some patients, or their significant others, may not even follow through all the five descriptors. Some people will relate to just one of the stages and not move to any of the others. The nursing associate should be able to recognise the stage(s) and what to expect when communicating with the person at each stage.

Denial

This is the initial coping mechanism for someone faced with news or a diagnosis that is so overwhelming it is difficult to understand and process. Denial allows the information to be absorbed slowly and lets the shock of that event or news to start to ease.

It is not uncommon for people to withdraw and appear numb or suggest that a mistake has been made and the information is wrong. Denial protects the body from the intense stress of a situation. If a person moves on from denial, then the healing process towards acceptance can begin.

Anger

Anger is often associated with phrases like 'why me?', 'It's not fair!', 'what did I ever do to deserve this?!' The anger can also be associated with a need to blame others for the cause of the emotional pain they are experiencing.

Expressing anger is a necessary stage of grief and is entirely understandable. They may be grieving for the loss of a loved one or for the loss of their future self if facing a life-limiting diagnosis. When a person feels grief, they feel abandoned and alone in an unfamiliar landscape of emotions. Expressing anger is a familiar emotion which helps ground the person to something real.

However, as much as anger is an important step in grief, it must not be left to get out of control. You do still need to be mindful of the need for de-escalation. Earlier in the chapter, you looked at de-escalation and the various communication techniques you can use. Many of those could also apply here.

Bargaining

Bargaining, in this context, is an act of desperation that is associated with guilt. It is associated with no end of 'what if' statements: 'what if I start eating five a day from now on', 'what if I had made the doctor's appointment earlier', 'what if I had left work five minutes earlier, the accident would not have happened'.

It is the process of trying to make sense of the situation.

Depression

Depression is the commonly expected emotion that is associated with dying and grief. It is where the person will withdraw emotionally, but they may also withdraw physically and distance themselves from others. They may struggle to get out of bed and not be interested in caring for themselves.

Depression is an exhausting state where the person will experience feelings of hopelessness and may even experience suicidal thoughts. This stage is by far the most dangerous for the individual.

Acceptance

For the significant others left behind after a death, acceptance is not the state of being okay that their wife has died. Rather, it is about knowing that their wife has died and that they are going to be okay. With acceptance, they enter a new state of reality and emotions start to become more stable. There are going to be good days and bad days, but as times goes on, the good days will outnumber the bad days. They will re-engage with friends and loved ones again as they adjust to the new reality.

For those patients with a life-limiting diagnosis, it is about finding peace in the time they have left.

Dying

There is a unique challenge that only applies when caring for the dying, where the family are requesting information be kept from the patient. Lawton and Carol (2005) called this the conspiracy of silence. In Activity 5.6, you will have an opportunity to think about how to manage this situation.

Activity 5.6   Critical thinking

You are working in the District Nursing team and have been called in to complete a pain assessment on a recently diagnosed palliative care patient. The patient's daughter greets you at the door and ushers you inside.

'Thank you for coming. Before I take you in to see Dad, I wanted to let you know that we, as a family, have decided that Dad must not know how ill he is. We know him best and we insist that you do not tell him. He would lose all hope and it would probably kill him!'

What are you going to do?

An outline answer is provided at the end of the chapter.

Activity 5.6 highlights how the denial of a terminal diagnosis and the fear of losing a loved one can influence behaviour.

Expressions of grief

The Kübler-Ross model outlines that there is no right or wrong way to grieve; it is unique to the individual. Likewise, there is no clear treatment for grief, neither is there a cure.

Grief can present itself in many ways and can be displayed as either a physical, social or spiritual expression, or as a combination of methods of expression. Crying would be the commonly expected expression of grief; however, some people do not have a natural ability to cry and will repress this emotion. This does not mean that they are not experiencing grief or that they don't care.

Many of the expressions associated with grief are also seen with stress in general, so worry, fatigue, an inability to sleep, loss of appetite and anxiety would be commonly seen and are driven by emotional responses. After the initial stress responses to the loss of a loved one, other emotions take over and the grieving person may express feelings of guilt, anger or frustration and may blame themselves for some aspect of the death.

Some will experience physical symptoms, such as muscular aches and pains, headaches or chest pain. The stress of grief can also induce flare-ups of stress-aggravated conditions, such as irritable bowel syndrome (IBS), psoriasis or eczema, and can make blood sugars unstable for those with diabetes.

Social expressions of grief are less obvious to healthcare professionals as these are often subtle changes that occur in the grieving person's home and social life and are brought about by a lack of communication, where no one wants to talk about the death. This often leads to isolation from friends and family and feelings of detachment.

Some people may also start to question spiritual aspects of life and the purpose of life. Now, this does not necessarily mean they are suicidal, questioning previously held beliefs or a want to become more spiritual in their life to feel closer to their lost loved one.

It is important to keep talking and giving the person experiencing grief the opportunity to express themselves and release the emotion associated with the situation they are in. Counselling and bereavement support groups can be very useful in helping the person work talk through their emotions and address the obstacles that grief creates in everyday life. Counselling does not remove the grief, but it does give strategies for coping with the grief.

Chapter summary

This chapter has explored the challenges that healthcare professionals may face when caring for people in heightened states of emotion. We have focused on the causes of aggression and violence and have discussed the use of de-escalation techniques.

We have also discussed the impact that conditions with mania and those that result in death, dying and grief have on communication in general. There have been opportunities to reflect on and explore contributing factors and the management of problems specific to those conditions.

Having the skills to manage situations of difficulty are very valuable tools in the nursing associate communication arsenal. It can make for a safer environment for staff, patients and the public, and can make the trauma of an incident more bearable and can give positive outcomes.

Activities: Brief outline answers

Activity 5.1 Critical thinking (page 79)

Physical health and general feelings of wellness impact on your mood, your ability to access services and therefore your behaviour. You may recall a time when you had a heavy cold and felt generally poorly, and that this had an impact on your mood and your behaviour. Similarly, with mental health, if you are feeling low in mood, then your physical behaviours will reflect that. These behaviours would contrast with what you display when you are feeling positive and confident.

There are experiences that are unique to an individual that will shape our behaviours and thought patterns, such as one's family structure and life experiences. Individual life experiences develop from a combination of cultural, societal or socioeconomic factors, your individual traits and your relationships with others.

Reflecting on your life experiences and comparing them to others around you and thinking about why people do what they do is a way to develop understanding for the uniqueness of those around you and to develop empathy, which will enhance your ability to communicate with all walks of life.

It may be that you come from a single-parent family living in a city, or you could have been brought up in a military family who moved around frequently. A comparison of country life to city life or living on a strict budget or having a large disposable income will all have an influence on what shapes a decision or behaviour.

This is not an exhaustive list.

Activity 5.2 Critical thinking (page 81)

Physical disorders related to conditions such as diabetes and infections can cause confusion, as can conditions that cause reduced oxygen uptake, leading to hypoxia, high temperatures and changes in the blood's acid base balance and changes in the blood flow to the brain or the deterioration in brain activity or cognitive ability.

Other factors that interfere with electrolytes within the body can also have an impact on confusion, such as urinary tract infections.

Factors associated with lifestyle choices and addictive behaviours, such as substance abuse disorders, including the excess use of alcohol, can cause confused states. These confused states may be temporary or may be as a result of prolonged exposure.

Mental health disorders can be assumed to be the major cause of confused states, but physical causes should not be dismissed if the patient has a prior mental health disorder diagnosis. There are many disorders that are commonly associated with delusions, hallucinations and confusion, such as dementia, bipolar disorders and psychosis.

This is not an exhaustive list.

Activity 5.3 Case study (page 82)

Warning signs of irritated or agitated behaviour could include:

- raised voices:
  - swearing
  - short, clipped answers to questions
- uncharacteristic silence
- sarcastic remarks:
  - mocking others

- negative body language:

  o threatening gestures such as finger pointing or foot stamping
  o pacing back and forth
  o crossed arms
  o aggressive posture, such as clenched fists

- negative facial expressions:

  o stare
  o frown
  o pursed lips/tight jaw/invade personal space

- aggressive behaviour:

  o slamming doors
  o kicking furniture or hitting themselves
  o throwing things

If patients are already known to you – inpatients on a psychiatric ward, for example – learn which triggers can result in violence and aggression for individuals, then work to avoid these.

This is not an exhaustive list.

Activity 5.4 Interprofessional team working (page 86)

1. What are your next steps?

You could end the call quickly and hang up. You can, after all, ring the bed manager back later. Go and investigate the situation.

2. What are your next steps and what is your priority?

It is clear that this situation needs an immediate de-escalation. The male patient is the priority. You need to safely move him away from the situation and calm him down. Approach him slowly, trying to get some eye contact and addressing him by name. Make sure you maintain an open posture and ask simple questions to distract the male patient away from the female patient and the HCSW.

Some example questions could be:

- '[Name of patient], what is upsetting you?'
- 'Can I help you get more comfortable?'

You will need to address the HCSW to call for assistance and get them to reassure the female patient in that order. Getting further assistance is vital to ensure the safety of the patients and staff.

3. What are your next steps?

Once in the bed space, draw the curtains around the male patient to maintain his dignity, but leave enough space so you can leave quickly if necessary and so that he can be observed discreetly by staff to ensure his safety.

Ask another member of staff to attend the female patient and relieve the HCSW. The HCSW may be upset and unnerved by what took place and would need time to compose themselves.

4. What would you say?

Starting communication after a frightening or upsetting event is important. The male patient likely feels confused and maybe embarrassed, which may leave him feeling vulnerable and isolated.

Using the skills of paraphrasing, brief commenting, the principle of the patient owning the problem and setting expectations, you will have the knowledge to prevent a repeat of the events.

- 'How are you feeling now?'
- 'I can understand that you were feeling confused and upset.'
- 'That must have been worrying for you.'
- 'I can understand why you were upset.'
- 'I wouldn't like to see you that upset again, so how can we make sure this doesn't happen again?'

5. What should happen now and what are you going to focus on?

For the staff involved in the incident, it is important that lessons are learned from the situation to avoid a reoccurrence. Using the NHS resolution 'Being Fair' (NHS Resolution, 2019), the debrief should not apportion blame in the events.

A good debrief should give a clear description of the events, including a timeline if possible. Personal reflection for those involved is to be encouraged as part of the debrief, as the HCSW should be able to reflect on the fact that standing with her hands on her hips can be seen as an aggressive stance. A debrief should also include a description of the environment and any possible triggers to the situation.

The debrief should come to some conclusions and recommendations for action to prevent a similar situation occurring again. It may be that the female and the male bays need to be swapped round, so the male patients are closer to the male toilet or there may be a need for clearer signage on the ward.

In addition to the debrief, there needs to be an incident report completed for the event and for injury to the HCSW, re the shoulder injury. The NA, as the accountable professional who delegated the task to the HCSW, has a duty of care towards the HCSW and needs to reflect on the incident and learn from mistakes made. A report should also be made in the patients' notes, identifying the triggers, causes and the actions taken (if any).

Activity 5.5 Reflection (page 88)

Research undertaken by Black and Curtis (2002) on communicating bad news to patients found that patients reported a variety of emotional reactions on hearing bad news. The study focused on a patient receiving a cancer diagnosis, where they recorded the most frequently expressed reactions: 54% of the patients felt in shock; 46% were afraid; 40% went directly to acceptance; 24% were sad; and 15% were 'not worried'.

How did this compare to your reflection?

The main issues seem to be regarding confusion and the patient misunderstanding the technical language. In a study involving 100 women with breast cancer, 73% did not understand the prognosis or the survivability information given to them by their doctors.

Activity 5.6 Critical thinking (page 93)

In a situation where you are being asked to withhold information from a patient, it is important to consider the reasons behind the request. It is likely that the family merely want to protect the patient from any further bad news and believe their relative would not be able to cope. Your first step is to acknowledge their concerns and explore the reasons behind the request.

While a patient has the mental capacity to understand and comprehend what is being told to them, they are entitled to information about their condition. There should not be a point, while caring for someone, that the family knows more about the patient's diagnosis than the patient, as long as the patient has mental capacity. Well-meaning family members should be advised that honesty is an essential part of the nurse–patient relationship. If they require reassurance, you can explain that nothing will be said that would directly harm the patient.

All good communication must be patient-led and driven by what the patient wants and needs. To be able to care for the person effectively relies on communication.

Knowledge review

Now that you have worked through the chapter, how would you rate your knowledge of the following topics?

	Good	Adequate	Poor
• communicating with people in heightened emotional states			
• de-escalating an angry communication			
• approaching difficult conversations			
• delivering empathic communication			
• understanding the causes of aggression and violence			

If you are unsure of some aspects, what are you going to do next?

Further reading and useful websites

For more information on how to prevent violent situations:
National Institute for Health and Care Excellence (NICE) (2015) *Costing Statement: Violence and Aggression. Implementing the NICE Guidelines on Violence and Aggression (NG10)*. Manchester, UK: National Institute for Health and Care Excellence.

For more information on the appropriate use of restraint:
www.nice.org.uk/guidance/ng10/chapter/1-Recommendations#anticipating-and-reducing-the-risk-of-violence-and-aggression-2

For more information on de-escalating angry situations:
Lowry, M. and Lingard, G. (2016) Deescalating anger: a new model for practice. *Nursing Times*, 112(4): 4–7.

More information on mental capacity, and the ability to make decisions, can be found in the Mental Capacity Act (2005):
www.legislation.gov.uk/ukpga/2005/9/contents

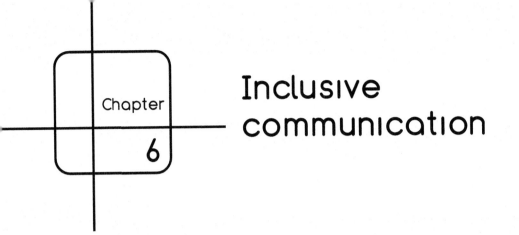

Inclusive communication

Chapter **6**

Annexe A: Communication and relationship management skills

At the point of registration, the nursing associate will be able to safely demonstrate the following skills:

2. Underpinning communication skills for providing and monitoring care:
1.8 be aware of the possibility of own unconscious bias in communication encounters.

Chapter aims

By the end of this chapter, you will be able to:

- understand the language and terms relating to diversity and equality.
- recognise the impact of the unconscious bias on communication.
- understand types and cause of discrimination.
- be aware of strategies for inclusive communication.
- consider the needs of the diverse populations.
- reflect on being able to challenge insensitive behaviour.

Introduction

The 2011 census recorded 63 million people within the United Kingdom, 8 million of whom registered as being from a minority ethnic background. Although, with the recent rise in popularity of home DNA testing to uncover our genealogical past, we can argue that the UK is even more diverse than we expect, with many different people coming together to form this island we call home.

Within this chapter, the focus is on communication, and the nature of diversity and equality will be discussed in line with the Equality Act's (2010) protected characteristics. We will explore the impact of conscious and unconscious biases to care provision and how to address insensitive behaviour.

To be able to intelligently apply communication skills which address inequalities and cultural sensitives with regards to the protection of others, we need, first, to understand what equality and diversity is, what the law says and how discrimination can be evident.

Diversity and equality

Diversity can be defined as the differences between people. It is the elements that make us unique, such as personality traits and how someone thinks. Diversity can also include aspects which define a person's identity, such as the shape of a person's body, ethnicity, age, gender, mobility or sexual orientation, to name a few.

Equality is about ensuring all the elements that make us diverse are accepted and no one trait, choice or aspect of that identity is measured more highly than another, or that one person takes precedence over another due to the aspect of a personal identity.

Protected characteristics and protection from discrimination

Under the law and the Equality Act (2010), we are protected from discrimination in the workplace, in education, as a customer or consumer, when using a public service, buying or renting a property and as a member or guest of a private club or association.

There are also certain characteristics that are protected under the Equality Act (2010). Specifically, there are nine characteristics. These are seen in Figure 6.1.

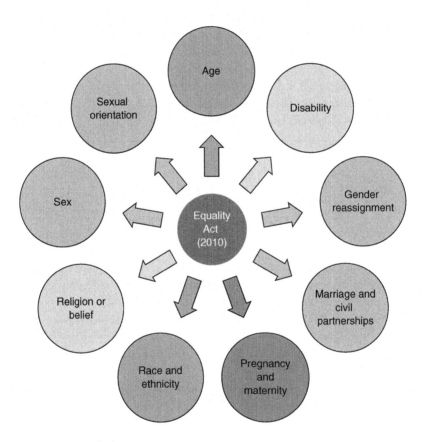

Figure 6.1   Protected characteristics.

Types of discrimination

There are seven types of discrimination that have been recognised by the Equality Act (2010). These are as follows.

Direct discrimination

This is where someone is treated less favourably than another person due to either a protected characteristic they have, a characteristic they are assumed to have or by association with someone with a protected characteristic.

An example would be a patient who is refused care on the basis that they are considered too old.

Indirect discrimination

This is where a policy, procedure, condition, rule or general working practice applies to everyone, but it has a significant impact on people with a protected characteristic. Indirect discrimination can be lawfully justified if it can be demonstrated that the action was reasonable and that there is a legitimate aim which has taken into account the least discriminatory route.

An unlawful example would be a manager who has changed the shift pattern for a ward, which means everyone works fewer but longer days. This new shift pattern discriminates against a member of staff with a disability that means that they have physical difficulties doing long days in practice. Where the disability is known by the manager, this could also be described as discrimination arising from a disability.

A lawful example, which is referred to as objective justification, could be where someone who has uncontrolled epilepsy needs to submit their driving licence and will not be permitted to drive. There are no reasonable adjustments that could be made to protect the driver or those around them, if they were to drive.

In addition to the lawful examples, there are sometimes occupational requirements, whereby a protected characteristic is required. For example, requiring female volunteers to help in a refuge for women, or needing a particular religious leader or minister to deliver a religious service.

Associative discrimination

Associative discrimination applies to all the protected characteristics and refers to discrimination due to knowing or being associated with someone who has a protected characteristic. For example, a mother of a child with a disability being refused flexible working hours so they can care for their child.

Discrimination arising from disability

This happens when someone is treated unfairly because of an issue arising from their disability. An example could be when someone with a known disability is dismissed or not offered a suitable alternative employment due to sickness relating to their disability.

Discrimination by perception

This is a form of direct discrimination against someone because others think they possess a protected characteristic. This applies whether they have the protected characteristic or not.

An example of this could be a nurse who is condescending and patronising towards a service user because they think they have a learning difficulty, or a shop worker who bullies a colleague they believe to be gay.

Harassment (inclusive of sexual harassment)

This is unwanted behaviour, which is felt by the recipient to be violating, offensive, intimidating, hostile and degrading, even if the behaviour is not directed specifically at them. Harassment does not have to involve physical contact; it can also be verbal, written or through gestures.

Victimisation

People can be subject to victimisation by being treated badly or unfairly if they have made or supported a complaint or grievance.

Now that we have identified some different types of discrimination, it is a good idea to consider how many you recognise and would be able to identify in practice. See Activity 6.1 for a scenario-based exploration of discrimination in practice.

Activity 6.1   Critical thinking

You are working in a busy inner-city GP surgery. There are multiple clinics going on and the waiting rooms are busy. Look at the sample interactions involving communication and decide which form of discrimination (if any) is in use in each of the examples.

1. A man approaches the reception desk and extends his hand to the receptionist to shake. She offers her hand as a greeting, but the man does not let go of her hand and uses his other hand to hold her wrist while he starts stroking her hand. He starts telling her how lovely she looks, and the receptionist is clearly uncomfortable.
2. The surgery uses a patient call system which flashes up the patient's name on a monitor screen with a short direction of which room they should go to for their appointment. Due to the busy nature of the medical centre, the names only appear for a few seconds before they disappear.
3. Sally has **macular degeneration** and is registered blind due to her visual impairment. The clinic is busy, and she could not get a seat close enough to the monitor screen to see her name clearly. Without realising, she missed her name and the appointment and has been recorded as DNA (did not attend). After waiting for a further 40 minutes, she approaches the reception desk to enquire about her appointment. She is told she was a DNA and that she needs to make another appointment. Sally explains that she had booked in, but the surgery policy is if a patient books in and does not attend within 30 minutes of the appointment where there is no surgery delay, they are assumed to have left the surgery and are recorded as DNA. Because Sally is recorded as DNA, she is told that the next appointment won't be available for two weeks and, furthermore, that surgery policy states that if she does not attend two appointments in a row, she will be removed from the surgery list.

4. Alannah and her friend Zuza sit together in the waiting room and talk in their native Romanian language. Zuza is there to see the midwife and, being heavily pregnant, goes to take a seat in the waiting space. Meanwhile, Alannah, who speaks very little English, books her friend in for the appointment with the midwife's administrative assistant. Another pregnant woman comes in and also books herself in with the administrative assistant. The assistant tells her she is 'going to fit her in before that foreign woman and make her wait. I don't think she should get free healthcare over here and she should go back home', while gesturing towards Zuza and Alannah. Zuza, who speaks excellent English, Romanian and German, overhears the conversation and turns to address the assistant, who ignores her. The assistant continues with 'I don't know why she is looking at me, it's not like she can understand me.'

An outline answer is provided at the end of the chapter.

In Activity 6.1, there was an opportunity to explore types of discrimination. It is important to note that discrimination manifests in many ways with enduring effects. For example, it can be a physical barrier, such as buildings only accessible to able-bodied people, or a barrier to employment when someone is refused an interview or job due to the colour of their skin or their gender identity. As the activity highlighted, discrimination can also occur through communication.

Communication is of central importance when considering the barriers caused by discrimination. Consider accessibility and the right to equal access. When people think about the word accessibility, they often think about ramps into a building, handrails and the use of lifts. Some may go so far as to recognise the need for private rooms to be available, for sensitive discussions to take place. Others may consider accessibility under the umbrella of Health and Safety and how we could evacuate someone with mobility issues from a building if there were a fire and the lifts cannot be used.

As much as those thoughts are correct, they fall short of inclusive communication. Inclusive communication starts with knowing who you are trying to communicate with. Is the issue a language barrier, or a hearing or sight deficit? The specifics of inclusive communication and communication tools are explored in more depth in Chapter 7.

Inclusive communication and the LGBTQIA+ community

We know that language matters and has power. It is a means of offering respect and understanding and acknowledging someone's identity. It is easy to make assumptions about a person's identity and this can cause offence, so, as nursing associates, use of inclusive communication is vital. When communicating with someone who identifies as being part of the LGBTQIA+ community, using inclusive language is important for empowering the individual. Let's now consider what this inclusive language looks like, in order to normalise the terms and minimise mistakes.

The acronym LGBTQIA+ captures different aspects of identity, which may include an individual's sexuality or sexual orientation, their gender identity, which is a social and psychological aspect of identity, and/or their sex, which is their biological identity. Figure 6.2 outlines which each letter in the LGBTQIA+ often refer to but it is important to remember that language is not fixed but constantly evolving. For a longer list of LGBTQIA+ terms, see the Stonewall website link at the end of the chapter. We explore the difference between gender and sex more below.

Lesbian	The term lesbian primarily relates to a woman who is sexually and/or romantically attracted to other women, or female same-sex relationships.
Gay	The term gay is currently more commonly associated with same-sex male relationships but can also be used for female same-sex relationships.
Bisexual	Bisexuality is a much-debated sexual identity and is often overlooked. It refers to someone who finds both men and women attractive, who may engage in relationships with people of the same or different sex or gender to themselves.
Trans	The term trans literally means the 'across' or opposite. In the context of trans people, the term relates to a gender identity that differs from their biological anatomical sex.
Queer or Questioning	The term 'queer' is still regarded as a derogatory or offensive term in many areas and should be used with caution. However, some individuals who feel that the terms lesbian, gay, bisexual or trans do not fully meet or explain their feelings about their sexuality and gender identity are repurposing the word as a descriptor. Q may also denote someone who is currently unsure of their sexuality and are exploring or questioning their sexual preferences.
Intersex	Intersex is a general term for people who are born with reproductive organs or sexual anatomy that does not fit into what would be considered typical for a male or female.
Asexual	Asexuality is when someone experiences little or no sexual attraction to others. This is different from celibacy, as celibacy is a choice.
+	The + symbol is an inclusive terms which represents other sexual identities, such as pansexual, bi-curious, gender fluid and others.

Figure 6.2   LGBTQIA+.

Sex and gender

Gender, in a broad sense, can be seen as the socially constructed characteristics that define someone as male or female. Sex, on the other hand, refers to the biological and anatomical structures that determine someone as a woman or a man. Where an individual's birth sex and gender identity align, they are referred to as 'cisgender'. The term 'trans' relates to an individual whose gender identity differs from their birth sex. As we have seen, gender is a social construct and some people may not feel they are either male or female, irrespective of their sex. These individuals may refer to themselves as non-binary (gender-neutral), bi-gender, a-gender, genderqueer or genderfluid.

Social transitioning

The social transition is when a trans person comes out to those around them. The social transition from one sex to another to align with a person's gender identity is a difficult process and is arguably more challenging than any medical or surgical intervention. Indeed, many trans people do not undergo such interventions. The transition can include a change in appearance and apparel and may involve the inclusion of a prosthesis or binding, which will change the contour of the body. Significantly, someone who has come out as trans may change their name. In terms of communication, using the correct name and the correct descriptor is essential in ensuring inclusion, dignity and respect. Once a name change has been announced, to use the birth or former name of the trans person is called 'dead naming'.

Within healthcare, there is a risk in using a dead name when addressing someone. When everyone is born, they are allocated an NHS number, which is linked to the person's birth name. If a person presenting outwardly as a female arrives at a general clinic, but their NHS number is associated with a male title and name, this does not mean there is an error or some misdealings.

In these instances, care needs to be taken to ensure you do not cause offence by using the dead name or by using gendered language. Gendered language makes reference to words we use that define a gender, such as: 'Mr and Mrs', 'ladies and gentlemen', 'boys and girls', 'brothers and sisters', 'policeman and policewoman', or even nursing Sister.

As a nursing associate and a competent communicator, it is important you are aware of and can use the correct pronouns for the people you are communicating with. In Activity 6.2, pronouns will be explained and the difference between binary and non-binary pronouns will be explored.

Activity 6.2 Work-based learning: pronouns and communication

Pronouns make up a small subcategory of nouns, which identify a person, a place, or a thing. The distinguishing aspect of a pronoun is that they can be substituted for other nouns. For example, if you're telling a story about your dog Sherman, the story will begin to sound repetitive if you keep saying 'Sherman' repeatedly. Consider the difference between these two examples:

Example 1: 'Sherman is my dog, and Sherman likes bones. Sherman has a special bone that Sherman likes to take to people when Sherman greets people in the house.'

Example 2: 'Sherman is my dog, and he likes bones. He has a special bone that he likes to take to people when he greets them in the house.'

The pronouns associated with people fall into two categories of either binary/ gendered or non-binary/gender-neutral. Commonly used gendered pronouns include she/her/hers and he/him/his, and commonly used gender-neutral pronouns include they/their/theirs. However, there are many more pronouns in use, some of which are explored in Figure 6.3 with their pronunciation in [' '].

(Continued)

(Continued)

1	2	3	4	5
Subject	Object	Possessive	Possessive Pronoun	Reflexive
Binary pronouns (gendered)				
he	him	his	his	himself
she	her	hers	hers	herself
Non-binary pronouns (gender neutral)				
e/ey ['e']	em ['m']	eir ['err']	eir	eirself ['err-self']
per	per	pers	pers	perself
they	them	their	theirs	themself
ve ['vee']	ver	vis ['viz']	vis	verself
xe ['zhee']	xem ['zhem']	xyr ['zhere']	xyrs ['zhers']	xemself ['zhem-self']
ze/zie ['zee']	zim	zir ['sir with a z']	zirs	zirself
Co	Co	cos ['coes']	cos	coself
hir ['here']	hir	hirs ['heres']	hirs ['heres']	hirself ['here-self']

Figure 6.3   Pronouns.

Complete the following sentences using a combination of some of the pronouns.

1. From the subject column (1): _____ laughed at the picture of a dog wearing a bow tie.
2. From the object column (2): The group tried to convince _____ to join them on an evening out.
3. From the possessive column (3): The large green armchair was _____ favourite place to read.
4. From the possessive pronoun column (4): The security guard asked if the red car parked out the front was _____.
5. From the reflexive column (5): The nursing associate was very pleased with _____ once the clinic had finished.

Now try this: practise using the different sets of pronouns in this short paragraph.

_____ (1) knew that _____ (2) blood pressure was high and that_____ (1) needed to take the medication the doctor has prescribed for _____(2), but _____(1) could not bring _____(5) to take it because the side effects sounded terrible. _____ (3) friend said to take medication and see how it goes, but the decision was _____(4) to make.

Outline answers are provided at the end of the chapter.

In Activity 6.2, we explored the use of pronouns to reflect sensitivity in communication with the LGBTQIA+ community. We will now move on to communication with other minoritised groups.

Communication and other minoritised groups

The United Kingdom is ethnically diverse, with people from a vast range of countries, cultures and religions. A commonly used umbrella term for those from minority ethnic communities is BAME, which should be pronounced as B-A-M-E and stands for Black, Asian and Minority Ethnic. The term BAME is problematic because it fails to distinguish between a multitude of different groups and communities, each with their own distinct experiences, challenges and identities. As such, caution should be exercised in using the term BAME and when referring or speaking to an individual, you should be appropriately specific. However, the term remains in frequent use in the NHS, in research and policy documents and many other contexts, and therefore it is important to understand.

A person's identity is made up of so much more than the colour of their skin, their ethnicity or nationality. It is important not to define any individual by a single characteristic, just as you wouldn't solely define a patient by their diagnosis. It is clear there is a need for cultural competence as a nursing associate. Cultural sensitivity in communication is about having the ability to be appropriately responsive to the attitudes, feelings or circumstances of groups of people or individuals that have a distinctive ethnic, national, religious, linguistic or cultural heritage (DHHS, OMH, 2001, p. 131, cited in Tucker et al., 2011).

The Covid-19 pandemic brought about a reality check on the need to improve health communication with minority ethnic groups, as shown by the lower-than-average uptake in the vaccination programme within these groups. The reliance on digital communication to provide information on the virus and how to access services and vaccination centres is often exclusionary. This is reflective of wider inequalities in access to health due to ethnicity. For example, Omer et al. (2020) comment that financial barriers around accessing digital data, a lack of internet connection and of devices, plus cultural and religious practices, all impact on the health of minority ethnic groups, along with difficulties in literacy, language and the ability to navigate information online.

In Activity 6.3, we shall explore some of the many languages that make up the population of the United Kingdom and consider what it is like to decipher a simple message in a language we don't understand.

Activity 6.3 Communication and multi-culturalism

Below are six examples of languages spoken within the United Kingdom. Each language is conveying the same message. Can you correctly identify the language, and can you decipher the message? If you already know one or more of the languages, choose one that is new to you.

1. नमस्ते मेरा नाम है (spoken as: namaste mera naam hai)
2. Buna numele meu este

(Continued)

(Continued)

3. こんにちは、私の名前は (spoken as: Kon'nichiwa, watashinonamaeha)
4. Cześć, mam na imię
5. Kamusta? Ang pangalan ko ay
6. สวัสดีฉันชื่อ (spoken as: S̄wạs̄dī c̄hạn chụ̄x)

Outline answers are provided at the end of the chapter.

Activity 6.3 highlights the richness of language but also the complexities of getting a simple message across that respects all cultures without discrimination.

Unconscious bias

As humans, we are hard wired to make snap judgements based on intuition and past experiences, which affects our attitudes or behaviours. These judgements happen so quickly we are not conscious or aware of them, and they will have a direct impact on the quality and nature of communication.

To understand this fully, we need to understand that there are three recognised states of mind. The first is the conscious brain, which defines and directs thoughts, action and awareness when we are actively aware of what we are thinking. An example of this would be if someone asked you whether you liked the food they served you to eat. Your brain acts like an internal search engine, focuses on the task and gives you options on how to respond. You then consciously choose the response.

Then, we have the subconscious brain, which acts as a filter for the information we are constantly receiving through our senses. It is responsible for filing away data received and, when called upon, can guide our actions and reactions. An example here would be when asked to recall your car's number plate or a friend's phone number. We know the information is there, but it is not needed in everyday use, so the subconscious brain has filed it. Another example of when the subconscious brain is effective is when we breathe. For most of the time, breathing is something we just do without the need for thought, as it is a **homeostatic** response. Although we can take control of it by engaging the conscious brain and focusing on wanting to take a deep breath, we override the subconscious brain. This is like when we do an activity that has been practised repeatedly and no longer requires conscious thought or actions.

Finally, we have the unconscious brain, which can be seen as the deep dark recesses of the mind. It is thought to have a key function in managing threats, helping us determine whether something is safe. The unconscious brain is in part linked to the Amygdala, which is in the temporal lobe of the brain **anterior** the hippocampus. The Amygdala is the structure responsible for recognising a threat. Once a threat is detected, it starts a hormonal response which stimulates the autonomic nervous system (ANS), triggering the **fight or flight response**. For example, if you have ever had food poisoning and been sick as a result, when you are presented with the same food that previously made you ill, the Amygdala will stimulate the responses in the body that will deter you from eating that food again, such as making you feel nauseous or other unpleasant feelings.

From the perspective of basic human survival, subconscious judgements or biases are necessary and, on occasion, essential. They become a problem when we allow these judgements to affect our behaviour in relation to the protected characteristics or in the context of it affecting the fair and equitable treatment of those in our care.

There are many recognised biases, some of which may be more obvious than others, and as a nursing associate, you must be able to recognise your biases and ensure that they do not affect care delivery in any way. Every person must be treated equally and fairly with no one person being seen as more or less important than another. The responsibilities of a nursing associate go beyond managing your own biases to checking and addressing the behaviour of others too. This will be explored in more detail in Chapter 9. To assist with understanding bias and the possibilities of discrimination, we will explore different biases.

Affinity bias

Where we are drawn to people who are similar, or share similar interests, backgrounds or experiences. Being biased towards people of similar experiences and opinions may mean that a person would likely 'fit in' to a group, but it limits diversity and inclusion. Choosing to spend more time talking to the person from your hometown, over someone who is not, is an example of an affinity bias.

Confirmation bias

This is almost a classic form of bias, where someone draws a conclusion about someone based on their personal experiences and does not see the other individual as an individual in their own right. If you think back to Activity 6.1, scenario 3, the HCSW was biased based on her experiences of people who could not speak English fluently, and she discriminated against Zuza as a result.

Attribution bias

This is another form of bias that is based on the false perception of another, similar to confirmation bias. Attribution bias comes from prior experience of dealing with an individual or from certain personal attributes. An example here could be if you see a white male walking down the road with hair shaved very close to his head, wearing heavy boots and turned up jeans with a football shirt on. You may assume that they are a football hooligan and that they are likely to be racist. That may not be the case at all, but there is an image projected in the media as a football hooligan and hooliganism is associated with racism, as we have seen in the 2021 football European Cup when England played Germany.

As much as we know, from earlier on in this chapter, that quick judgements are part of being human, we need to consciously 'check' our biases to avoid prejudiced labels so we can effectively communicate.

Conformity bias

A conformity bias can also be seen as peer pressure. For example, when someone acts in a way that is not true to who they are or what they feel or believe, but as a means to fit in or be influenced by others. When considering communication, it is important to be mindful that patients are often influenced to conform. When they are admitted as inpatients, they conform to behaviours which they expect an inpatient or a sick person should demonstrate. This is referred to as 'the sick role' and first identified by American sociologist Talcott Parson in the 1950s (Frank, 2012). They can also be influenced by people whom they consider to be an authority and they will tell a healthcare professional what they think they want to hear rather than what they really feel. We will explore this point more with the authority bias.

Halo/horns effect

This is a bias based on placing someone in a position of high esteem. An example of this is celebrity culture. If a person perceives a celebrity as attractive and successful, they will also believe them to be likeable, intelligent, kind and funny. This can be linked to the bias on beauty attractiveness, whereby to be beautiful is to be good. In contrast, to be viewed as ugly would imply the person is not likeable.

The horns effect contrasts with the halo effect, where someone is judged negatively based on an actual or perceived unfavourable aspect about them.

Contrast effect

The contrast effect is about drawing comparisons and drawing conclusions from the differences or similarities between the objects being compared.

For example, if a patient on your ward finds you easier to talk to than your colleague, they are likely to show a bias in wanting to speak to you in comparison to your colleague.

Gender bias

Gender bias is based on the protected characteristic as outlined in the Equality Act (2010), where someone displays a preference towards a particular gender over another. We only need to look at the nursing profession to see this. Nursing and healthcare delivery has always had strong associations with women. In nursing, 90% of the workforce is made up of women. Women in the nursing workforce earn 17% less than their male counterparts. Furthermore, nurses with BAME origins on average earn 10% less than their white counterparts (RCN, 2020a).

Foss (2002), whose research focuses on age-related biases, suggests that, to some degree, gender bias is reflected in care delivery. Research conducted on patient satisfaction surveys noted that young female patients were less content with their care in comparison to young male patients. Female patients felt that the nurses were less caring and less committed to their care, that they had less time for them and that they lacked skill.

Ageism

Ageism is another bias associated with a protected characteristic, where someone is treated unfairly due to their age. This can happen at any age and is often a factor in healthcare decisions. If we consider the cervical screening (smear test) programme, a woman is only eligible for screening once they reach 25 years old. The screening is in main to check for changes in the cells on the cervix which could indicate possible cancers. The development of cervical cancer is associated with unprotected sexual intercourse and the Human Papillomavirus (HPV). This is a common virus for which there are over 100 types; two of those types are responsible for over 70% of all cervical cancers (WHO, 2020). If we, then, consider that the average age of a female in the UK losing their virginity is 18 years old (Palmer et al., 2019), to deny them access to cervical screening for seven years could be considered ageism.

However, the screening service is not intended to be discriminatory. It is associated with the average risk of developing cervical cancer and the cost of the screening service.

Name bias

The name bias is to judge someone on their actual or perceived background and personality based on their name. A recent example of a name bias is with the name 'Karen'. The name Karen has embedded itself in slang language because of common internet memes, and it has come to represent an entitled white woman demanding special treatment or favours, who is using their privilege to get their own way.

Names are like a label which sets an expectation that is often brought about from previous experiences of people with a similar name. An unfamiliar name makes the person unfamiliar. An androgenous name, which can be given to either gender, can lead to false expectations of the person.

Physical appearances bias (height, weight, physical disability, beauty/attractiveness)

To judge someone on their physical appearance, either negatively or as a favourable trait, is a bias. The bias against a physical disability is clear because it is represented in the Equality Act (2010) protected characteristics. Height and weight are not protected by the Equality Act, but there have been recent calls for them to be included as more and more legal cases claiming discrimination based on height and weight are seen by the court.

Aspects of some physical characteristics may need to be applied to some jobs, for the sake of safety and ability to perform the role. However, if a reasonable adjustment can be made to facilitate that person doing the job, then those measures should be taken. If reasonable adjustments can be made and they are not done, and by default the person does not get the job, then this is discrimination.

Anchor bias

An anchor bias is when a person relies too much on a single source of information or pre-existing information. The person is essentially 'anchored' to this position and will not move. This can be more clearly understood when we describe a person who says phrases like 'well, we always do it this way' or 'when I worked on my previous ward, we did...' These people are anchored to the past and will need some guidance to move forward. This will be explored in more depth in Chapter 9.

Being aware of the possible biases can help you understand what motivates some people and can help you apply theory to practice in order to address a bias in the future.

Chapter summary

This chapter has looked at equality and diversity with a focus on minority groups within the United Kingdom and how you as nursing associates can advocate for those in your care. It has explored the challenges faced by minority groups and those with protected characteristics. More importantly, it has outlined the theory around types of discrimination and unconscious biases that impact on behaviour and inclusion. As you move forward through this book, you will need the knowledge gained in this chapter to enhance your practice and allow you to celebrate the differences in the people you meet and enjoy the richness of the population.

Activities: Brief outline answers

Activity 6.1 Critical thinking (page 104)

Suggested answer 1: This is harassment. The man is being inappropriate, and the receptionist is feeling uncomfortable. If you were witness to this, it would be appropriate to step in and offer assistance to the receptionist and ask that the man release her. If he does so immediately, suggest the receptionist move back to a safer space. If he failed to comply with the request, the instruction to release her can become a demand. Policies for violence prevention and reduction should be reviewed.

Suggested answer 2: There are two aspects here. The first is indirect discrimination, where a policy or system negatively impacts on someone with a protected characteristic. In Sally's case, her sight is a disability and is as such protected. The GP system for announcing appointments does not work for someone with Sally's disability, unless she could sit closer to the screen, but no seats close to the screen have been secured for those with a disability. Second, the GP policy is detrimental to Sally. Reasonable adjustments in this case could be made, so the discrimination is unlawful. Also, Sally is subject to discrimination arising from a disability, the fact that she cannot see the screen, which leaves her at a disadvantage and being treated unfairly. More efforts should be made to use inclusive forms of communication.

Suggested answer 3: Like Sally's example in number 2, there are two forms of discrimination here. The first is direct discrimination: race and ethnicity is a protected characteristic and Zuza is being treated unfairly. Second, there is discrimination by association. The association aspect is because the assistant assumed that Zuza could not speak English because she was talking in Romanian to her friend, whose English was limited. It would be easy to see that pregnancy and maternity as a protected characteristic should be included in this discussion, but in this instance, Zuza is not being discriminated against due to being pregnant.

Activity 6.2 Work-based learning: communication and gender diversity (page 107)

1. From the subject column (1): _ve_ laughed at the picture of a dog wearing a bow tie.
2. From the object column (2): The group tried to convince _zim_ to join them on an evening out.
3. From the possessive column (3): The large green armchair was _eir_ favourite place to read.
4. From the possessive pronoun column (4): The security guard asked if the red car parked out the front was _hirs_.
5. From the reflexive column (5): The nursing associate was very pleased with _coself_ once the clinic had finished.

_Xe_ (1) knew that _xem_ (2) blood pressure was high and that _xe_ (1) needed to take the medication the doctor has prescribed for _xem_ (2), but _xe_ (1) could not bring _xemself_ (5) to take it because the side effects sounded terrible. _Xyr_ (3) friend said to take medication and see how it goes, but the decision was _xyrs_ (4) to make.

Activity 6.3 Communication and multi-culturalism (page 109)

Below are six examples of languages spoken within the United Kingdom. Each language is conveying the same message. Can you correctly identify the language, and can you decipher the message?

1. नमस्ते मेरा नाम है (spoken as: namaste mera naam hai): this is Hindi.
2. Buna numele meu este: this is Romanian.
3. こんにちは、私の名前は (spoken as: Kon'nichiwa, watashinonamaeha): this is Japanese.
4. Cześć, mam na imię: this is Polish.
5. Kamusta? Ang pangalan ko ay: this is Filipino.
6. สวัสดีฉันชื่อ (spoken as: S̄wạs̄dī c̄hạn chụ̄x): this is Thai.

The message each language is expressing is: 'Hello, my name is…'

Knowledge review

Now that you have worked through this chapter, how would you rate your knowledge of the following topics?

	Good	Adequate	Poor
• the terms which are used in diversity and equality cultures			
• the impact of unconscious bias on communication			

	Good	Adequate	Poor
• types and cause of discrimination			
• strategies for inclusive communication			
• the needs of diverse populations			
• challenging insensitive behaviour			

If you are unsure of some aspects, what are you going to do next?

Further reading and useful websites

For more on diversity and culture awareness in the nursing profession:
Brathwaite, B. (2020) *Diversity and Cultural Awareness in Nursing Practice.*
London: SAGE.

Transgender guide for NHS acute hospital trusts:
**http://s3-eu-west-1.amazonaws.com/files.royalfree.nhs.uk/E_and_D/
trasngender_booklet_low_res.pdf**

To learn more about health inequalities affecting people with learning difficulties,
please read the Death by Indifference Report by Mencap:
**www.mencap.org.uk/sites/default/files/2016-08/Death%20by%20Indifference%20
-%2074%20deaths%20and%20counting.pdf**

If you want to explore more about what unconscious biases you may have, visit the
Harvard University Project Implicit, which has a wide range of test and activities
that helps you uncover your unconscious biases:
https://implicit.harvard.edu/implicit/takeatest.html

Additional useful website

Stonewall, an LGBT rights charity based in the UK, has put together an extensive
list of LGBTQIA+ terms and descriptions:
**https://www.stonewall.org.uk/help-advice/faqs-and-glossary/list-lgbtq-
terms**

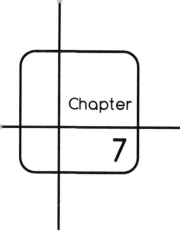

7

Communicating with patients who have specialist requirements

NMC FUTURE NURSE STANDARDS OF PROFICIENCY FOR NURSING ASSOCIATES

This chapter will address the following platforms and proficiencies:

Platform 1: Being an accountable professional

At the point of registration, the nursing associate will be able to:

1.11 provide, promote, and where appropriate advocate for, non-discriminatory, person-centred and sensitive care at all times. Reflect on people's values and beliefs, diverse backgrounds, cultural characteristics, language requirements, needs and preferences, taking account of any need for adjustments.

Platform 3: Provide and monitor care

At the point of registration, the nursing associate will be able to:

3.4 demonstrate the knowledge, communication and relationship management skills required to provide people, families and carers with accurate information that meets their needs before, during and after a range of interventions.

Annexe A: Communication and relationship management skills

At the point of registration, the nursing associate will be able to safely demonstrate the following skills:

1. Underpinning communication skills for providing and monitoring care:

    1.3 use appropriate non-verbal communication including touch, eye contact and personal space.

    1.12 recognise the need for translator services and material.

    1.13 use age-appropriate communication techniques.

(Continued)

(Continued)

2. Communication skills for supporting people to prevent ill health and manage their health challenges:

    2.3   use appropriate materials, making reasonable adjustments where appropriate to support people's understanding of what may have caused their health condition and the implications of their care and treatment.

    2.5   recognise and accommodate sensory impairments during all communications.

    2.6   support and monitor the use of personal communication aids.

    2.8   identify the need for and manage a range of alternative communication techniques.

Chapter aims

By the end of this chapter, you will be able to:

*   understand what is meant by the term 'sensory impairment'.
*   be able to consider the use of alternative communications tools which are age appropriate.
*   be able to consider the use of alternative communications tools that are cognitively appropriate.
*   explore the use and application of braille, British Sign Language (BSL) and Makaton.
*   understand what inclusive communication is.

Introduction

It is estimated that 2.2 million people in the UK regularly use alternative communication aids, but this does not include the 12 million with hearing impairments (Royal National Institute for Deaf people (RNID), 2018) or the millions of people who use glasses, contact lenses and hearing aids as part of their daily activities to assist in communication. Within this chapter, we will explore what sensory impairment is, and this will be broken down into hearing, visual, speech and verbalisation and the physical impairments that impact on communication. There is an opportunity to explore some communication techniques, with reference made to some specific conditions. Finally, this chapter will consider the principles of inclusive communication.

Sensory impairment

There are almost 2 million people within the UK living with some degree of sight loss and, of those, 360,000 are registered blind (NHS, 2018). There are 12 million people living with hearing loss, 151,000 of them use British Sign Language (BSL), with 87,000 being registered as deaf. Tinnitus affects 7.1 million people.

Tinnitus is a buzzing, hissing, whistling or ringing in both ears when there are no external sounds making those noises. It can be either a constant or intermittent sound which can vary in volume (British Tinnitus Association, 2021).

From looking at data from just two of our senses, we can see that from a population of roughly 65 million in the UK, 32% have a sensory impairment of either hearing or sight.

Sensory impairment goes further than hearing and sight. It includes taste, touch and smell. Outside of those senses, we rely on our balance and movement, via the vestibular system in the inner ear and through proprioception (also called **kinaesthesia**), which is the sense of self movement of the body and is in relation to the environment and spatial awareness (Martinez, 2019). For the purposes of communication, we will focus on hearing, slight and verbal/speech impairments or impediments. We must also be mindful of biomedical conditions like autism spectrum disorders and sensorineural hearing loss, as well as developmental language delays, which can contribute to communication impairments.

Hearing

Hearing impairments fall into three categories (see Figure 7.1), sensorineural, where there is damage to the tiny hair cells called stereocilia that are found in the inner ear. Or there is damage to the auditory nerve that leads from the ear to the brain. This kind of damage is permanent and irreversible (Tanna et al., 2021). The second category is a with a problem of sound conduction, which is where there is an obstruction or damage to the middle or outer ear that prevents sounds reaching the inner ear (Sooriyamoorthy and De Jesus, 2021). These are often temporary. The removal of the foreign body or ear wax and the treatment of any infection should rectify the problem. Mixed causes of hearing impairment are when a conductive problem meets with a sensorineural problem. For example, if you have hearing degeneration from ageing, and this is combined with impacted ear wax, the result could be a significant reduction in hearing or the loss of hearing altogether. Some aspects of a mixed hearing loss can be resolved.

There is a general assumption that an impairment means the loss of function or acuity of a sense, but in some cases that are associated with learning difficulties or an autistic spectrum disorder, there can be a hypersensitivity to noise. The individual in these cases

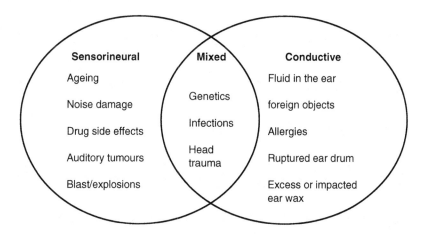

Figure 7.1 Types of hearing loss and their causes.

may wear noise-cancelling or noise-reducing ear defenders. These are intended to help reduce sensory overload (Bogdashina, 2014).

Regardless of the cause of the hearing impairments, we must focus on how we communicate. For the longer-term issues, once a full assessment of the problem that considers the age and developmental stage of the person is established, and the cognitive ability is confirmed, a range of options for communication is available.

The simplest form of communication would be through the written or typed word; however, there are physical aids to enhance hearing, such as hearing aids and the more advanced bone-anchored hearing aids (BAHA), as well as Bonebridge and Cochlear implants using bone vibration/conduction technology for hearing (Alzhrani, 2019).

Hearing aids and implants are not always a solution to hearing impairments, and as much as they do help with hearing, they cannot easily filter out the surrounding noises, so listening to one person speaking in a busy environment can still be difficult. Many shops and public service offices have an audio induction loop system or hearing loop installed. The loop system availability is indicated by the symbol in Figure 7.2

Figure 7.2 Audio induction loop symbol.

The loop system works by generating a magnetic field which, when the hearing aid is set to the 'T' position, helps reduce the extraneous noise from around the wearer and helps them hear speech with less disruption. The loop device can be a small box which sits neatly on a desk or counter space and can also be used to cover a room, such as a cinema auditorium or lecture theatre.

In the instances that the technological aids do not resolve a hearing impairment, but do allow the wearer to feel less vulnerable in public, other communication and support aids can be used to complement the hearing aid. Hearing dogs are an amazing companion animal for the hearing impaired. They reduce the social isolation and vulnerability often felt by the hearing impaired, help raise the alarm when an alarm cannot be heard, and they help to promote independence.

Another complementary mechanism for supporting communication with people with hearing impairment, but also impairments with speech and verbalisation, is the use of sign language(s).

Makaton is one form of sign language which uses hand signing. Some speech and symbols on communication cards are also used to communicate. It is a particularly useful form of communication with children because it can support the development of early years communication skills. It is also very useful with individuals with cognitive impairments, from autism to a range of other neurological disorders, including post-stroke rehabilitation and patients with dementia (Makaton.org, undated).

For those with long-term verbalisation issues, there is an option to develop a communication passport. The communication passport is a person-centred document that helps the reader understand more about the passport holder. It outlines their likes and dislikes, and it allows the holder to use images and words in their passport to communicate their wishes. In Activity 7.1, you will have the opportunity to review and address a section of a health passport (see Figure 7.3).

Activity 7.1   Work-based learning

Brandon is a 19-year-old person who has an autistic spectrum disorder. Brandon's disorder is associated with selective **mutism** due to a pronounced **stammer**. Brandon is due to have two impacted wisdom teeth removed as a day case patient.

1. Review the section of Brandon's health passport included here and describe what actions you would put in place to address Brandon's needs while in the day surgery department.
2. Immediately after the procedure, Brandon will be a little sleepy and not able to use the tablet device to communicate. You will need to use the communication book and the picture in it. Think about what pictures in Brandon's communication book would be relevant.

COMMUNICATION				Health passport 2021/2022			
Name	Brandon Kennedy	**Pronoun**	They		**Like to be called**	Brandon or Brandy	
How I would like you to communicate with me							
Involving someone else	Easy to read information		Communication book	x		Pictures	x
Drawing	Signing/Makaton		Signing and talking			Speaking directly to me	x
Looking me in the face	Smiling kindly		Speaking loudly			Gentle tone	
Using simple language	Other: Brandon needs to wear glasses	x	Other: With Augmentative and Alternative Communication (AAG) device (smart tablet)	x		Other: Be patient and give Brandon time to communicate	x

(Continued)

121

(Continued)

How I will communicate with you							
Tablet device	x	Communication book	x	Pictures	x	Simple hand gestures	x

Notes
I do not like to engage with eye contact for very long and will need my glasses to make sure I can see your faces clearly.
I prefer to use my tablet device to communicate but will use the communication book and pictures if they are not available. I am able to speak and make sounds, but I only do this freely when I am with people I am familiar with and trust.
I can understand what you are saying and as long as I have my glasses, I can read information well.

Things I would like to do that will help me be happy while in hospital.
I like to look at my magazines
Having my glasses on and being able to see what is happening
Being able to use my communication aids
Being able to contact Jackie if I feel anxious (my care worker) tel: 04778911546

Things I don't like that would make me feel sad in hospital.
Loud and sudden noises
Not having my glasses
Being in pain/distress: I will show distress by wringing my hands together repeatedly.
Not having a call bell
Not having my communication tools with me
Not being allowed to look through my magazines
Being kept in a room on my own
Being cold
Not being able to see Jackie (my care worker) tel: 0123456789
Shouting

Figure 7.3 Brandon's Health Passport.

Suggested answers can be found at the end of this chapter.

In Activity 7.1, we have introduced the use of the health passport for communication. The health passport is a very detailed document that covers many of a person's activities of daily life and is an important tool when caring for someone with communication problems. For more information on this, please refer to the useful website section at the end of this chapter.

The most recognised form of sign language is BSL. BSL shares many similarities with Makaton, when wishing to identify items, objects, places, feelings and emotions. Where BSL differs is with the addition of the finger spelling alphabet, which allows for complex iterations and descriptions. The following section explores the use of BSL and introduces you to the finger spelling alphabet.

Hello, my name is...

'Hello' (see Figure 7.4) is expressed by raising one of your hands to shoulder height, palm facing outwards and front facing with the fingers spread in a natural position. The hand is waved in a small arc left and right. It is important to speak out loud or mouth the word 'Hello', as the same gesture can be used for goodbye.

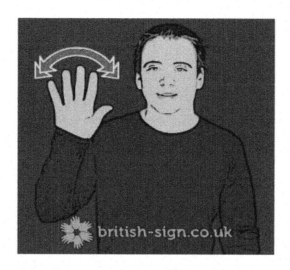

Figure 7.4   Hello.

Published with the kind permission of British-sign.co.uk.

The word 'my' (see Figure 7.5) is communicated by either hand being formed into a loose fist and the thumb tucked into the fist. This fist is then placed against the centre (middle) of the chest.

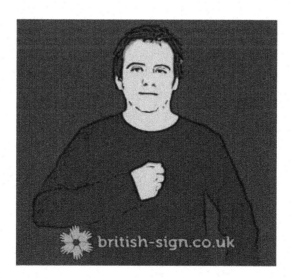

Figure 7.5   My.

Published with the kind permission of British-sign.co.uk.

For 'name', in Figure 7.6, you need to refer to Figure 7.7 and look for the symbol for 'N'. Form the letter 'N' and place the pads of the two extended fingers onto your forehead above the eye of the same hand you are using. So, if you have made the 'N' with your left hand, the pads of the extended fingers should be on your forehead over your left eye. To complete the word, you need to maintain the 'N' symbol, raising the fingers off your forehead slightly and keeping the hand at forehead height. Turn your hand at the wrist by pivoting the wrist away from you to essentially show the pads of the extended fingers to the reader of your sign language.

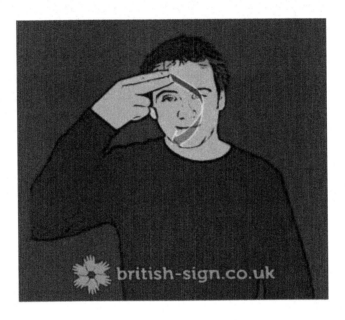

Figure 7.6   Name.

Published with the kind permission of British-sign.co.uk.

You would then, by referring back to Figure 7.7, spell and mouth out your name. In Activity 7.2, there is an opportunity for you to practise finger spelling your name in BSL.

Activity 7.2   Work-based learning: BSL practice

Having seen how to say 'Hello, my name is' in BSL, it is important that you can say your name in BSL. Please see Figure 7.7 below and practise spelling your name.

For more information on different signs and more activities using BSL, please see the useful websites section at the end of this chapter.

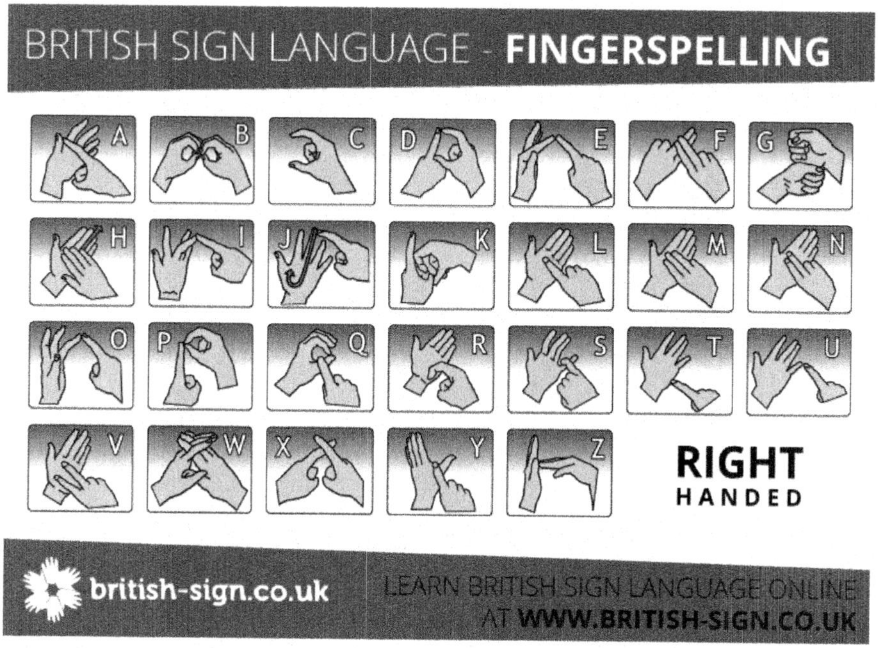

BRITISH SIGN LANGUAGE - **FINGERSPELLING**

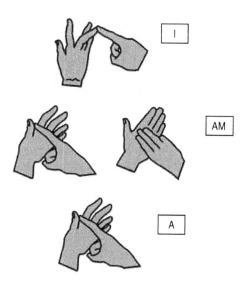

Figure 7.7   Finger spelling.

Published with the kind permission of British-sign.co.uk.

No outline answers are available for this activity.

You may also wish to communicate that you are a nursing associate. The universal sign of a nurse (see Figure 7.9) would be sufficient initially, but you may be required to stipulate the different role using the finger-spelling chart to spell out 'associate'. The start of the introduction in BSL can be seen in Figure 7.8.

Figure 7.8   I am a.

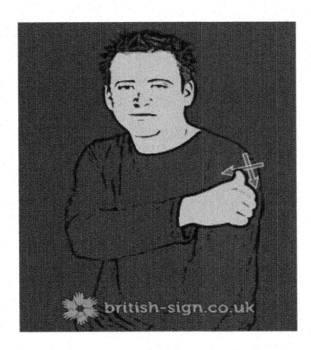

Figure 7.9   Nurse.

Published with the kind permission of British-sign.co.uk.

Sight

Impairments in sight or visual disruptions tend to fall into three categories: early years development, mixed and acquired (see Figure 7.10). The first and most difficult to predict are issues related early years development, which includes prenatal (before or at the point of conception), perinatally, which is from 28 weeks gestation through to the fourth week following a child's birth and postnatally, or conditions that develop after birth, but usually in infancy (Gogate et al., 2011).

Postnatally, and as part of the mixed causes for visual impairment, the child is at risk from Keratomalacia, which is caused by vitamin A (Retinol) deficiency. Vitamin A is found in red, yellow and orange fruits and vegetables. These are high in beta-carotene. It is also found in eggs, dairy products and dark green leafy vegetables. The most common cause of blindness in the developing countries is associated with vitamin A deficiency and the development of measles keratitis resulting in blindness. It is thought that measles causes 60,000 cases of blindness annually (Dang, 2015). Measles keratitis affects the cornea of the eye, but measles can attack any part of the eye, causing damage (Dang, 2015). Ensuring access to the Mumps, Measles and Rubella (MMR) vaccine is essential to prevent this cause of blindness, but inequalities in health and misinformation on the efficacy of vaccines means these conditions remain.

Along with eye diseases and disorders, the main cause of visual impairment comes from refractive errors. Refractive errors are a type of visual problem which makes it difficult to clearly focus on an object. Refractive errors occur when the shape of the eye prevents light reaching the retina, at the back of the eye. These errors cannot be prevented but are easily diagnosed by a trip to an optician for an eye examination, and they are easily treated with contact lenses or glasses.

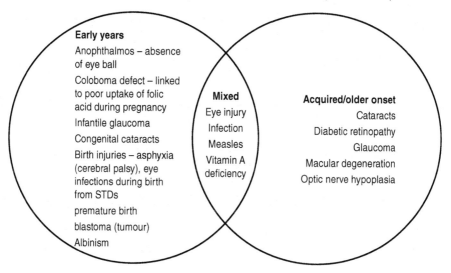

Early years

Anophthalmos – absence of eye ball

Coloboma defect – linked to poor uptake of folic acid during pregnancy

Infantile glaucoma

Congenital cataracts

Birth injuries – asphyxia (cerebral palsy), eye infections during birth from STDs

premature birth

blastoma (tumour)

Albinism

Mixed

Eye injury

Infection

Measles

Vitamin A deficiency

Acquired/older onset

Cataracts

Diabetic retinopathy

Glaucoma

Macular degeneration

Optic nerve hypoplasia

Figure 7.10 Causes of sight impairment.

The four common refractive errors are:

- myopia (near-sightedness): difficulty in seeing distant objects clearly;
- hyperopia (far-sightedness): difficulty in seeing close objects clearly;
- astigmatism: distorted vision resulting from an irregularly curved cornea, which is the clear covering front of the eye;
- presbyopia: which leads to difficulty in reading or seeing at arm's length. It is linked to ageing and occurs to almost everyone.

(WHO, 2013)

With respect to communication, the simplest course of action is to make sure that the person you are talking to has access to the aids they need to optimise their communication and decrease their feelings of vulnerability, such as making sure they are wearing their glasses or lenses and that they are clean and fit for purpose. In addition, there are spoken word documents, audio books, print readers, large print options and software that is voice activated and uses voice recognition to allow for the user to write/dictate. Being visually impaired is an isolating condition, which can make people feel vulnerable, so, like assistance dogs for the deaf, there are assistance dogs for the blind and visually impaired too. This allows the sufferer to maintain their independence and offers security and companionship.

In the next section, you will have an opportunity to explore the use of the oldest form of assistance for the visually impaired.

Braille alphabet

Braille was invented in 1824 by Louis Braille. He designed a system of using a combination of raised dots in a set of six that is used by visually impaired people to read and write. The system uses a different pattern for each letter of the alphabet (see Figure 7.11), some common words and instructions for the reader.

A (1)	B (2)	C (3)	D (4)	E (5)	F (6)	G (7)	H (8)	I (9)	J (0)
●○ ○○ ○○	●○ ●○ ○○	●● ○○ ○○	●● ○● ○○	●○ ○● ○○	●● ●○ ○○	●● ●● ○○	●○ ●● ○○	○● ●○ ○○	○● ●● ○○
K	**L**	**M**	**N**	**O**	**P**	**Q**	**R**	**S**	**T**
●○ ○○ ●○	●○ ●○ ●○	●● ○○ ●○	●● ○● ●○	●○ ○● ●○	●● ●○ ●○	●● ●● ●○	●○ ●● ●○	○● ●○ ●○	○● ●● ●○
U	**V**	**W**	**X**	**Y**	**Z**	**and**	**for**	**of**	**the**
●○ ○○ ●●	●○ ●○ ●●	○● ●● ○●	●● ○○ ●●	●● ○● ●●	●○ ○● ●●	●● ●○ ●●	●● ●● ●●	●○ ●● ●●	○● ●○ ●●
Capital letter	**To capitalise a whole word**								
○○ ○○ ○●	○○ ○○ ○●	○○ ○○ ○●							

Figure 7.11 Braille alphabet.

Braille is commonly used and can be found on many household products, particularly cleaning products and medicines. It can also be found in public signage and road crossings. In Activity 7.2, you can have a go at reading braille.

Activity 7.2 Work-based learning: braille and visual impairment

Referring back to Figure 7.11, can you read the following five braille examples (see Figures 7.12, 7.14, 7.15, 7.16 and 7.17.)?

1.

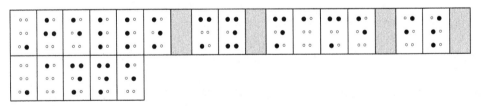

Figure 7.12 Braille example 1.

For numbers, a special character is placed before a letter which is used to represent a number. The special character is displayed in Figure 7.13. Following this special character, A would be used to represent number 1 and B would be used for number 2 and so on, all the way up to I which represents number 9. For zero, J in the alphabet is used (see Figure 7.11 for more information).

2.

Figure 7.13 Braille character to indicate a number.

Obviously, numbers are very important in the role of a nursing associate. Have a go at the next phrase and some number exercises.

3.

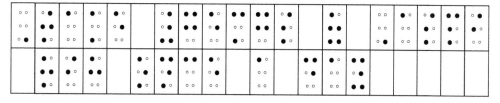

Figure 7.14 Braille example 3.

4.

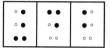

Figure 7.15 Braille example 4.

5.

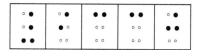

Figure 7.16 Braille example 5.

6.

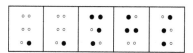

Figure 7.17 Braille example 6.

Answers to the questions are provided at the end of the chapter.

Activity 7.2 introduced the application of braille in communication. Now, look at those household products and the signs in the environment that contain braille and use the skills you have acquired with the activity to take time to work out what they say.

Physical impairments

As much as sign language and braille are very useful tools for those with visual and hearing impairments, these tools cannot be used for individuals with visual, hearing or verbalisation impairments when combined with physical impairments, where the arms and the hands either lack the sensitivity or the range of movement to use those tools.

In these instances, there are a range of devices that can be used to help with communication. There are low-tech options which use a board of common words and symbols that the user can use eye movements to point to, or a range of pointers that can be mounted on the head, in the mouth or adapted for use according to the needs of the person. In the further reading section at the end of this chapter, there is a link to the Mouth and Foot Painting Artists Association. Access the link to see an impressive collection of art produced using an artist's feet or mouth.

Technology, however, has made communication considerably more accessible. The pointers can be used on computer keyboards, and some come with a stylus for use on touch-screen devices. There is facial recognition software that will detect controlled movements of the face to aid in spelling out words and generating an electronic voice. The famous theoretical physicist, cosmologist and author Professor Stephen Hawking had Amyotrophic Lateral Sclerosis (ALS), which is a progressive neurological disease that leads to loss of muscle control. In the advanced stages of the disease, Professor Hawking used a computer screen that focused on the controlled movement of his cheek to write and converse.

With the development in technology, there are also considerable developments in augmented and alternative communication devices that can be adapted to users' needs. There is also a range of accessibility software that uses smart devices and computers, and which is suitable for use with any impairment that impacts communication.

Laryngectomy and tracheostomies

A laryngectomy is a partial or complete surgical removal of the larynx or voice box. This is usually as a result of laryngeal cancer.

With a complete laryngectomy, the entire larynx is removed and the trachea (windpipe) is brought up and out through the skin of the throat to form a stoma or hole, which will be permanent. This is referred to as a tracheostomy and it is through this hole that the person will breathe.

People with tracheostomies for other reasons outside of a laryngectomy will also be unable to make sounds even if their larynx is present. It is the breath passing through the larynx and over the vocal cords which makes sound and speech possible. The tracheostomy bypasses the larynx to allow air to go directly into the trachea and bronchi via the stoma (hole) in the throat.

In both instances, the connection between the throat and the oesophagus (food pipe) is not usually interrupted and food and liquids can be consumed as normal.

With a laryngectomy, it is possible to vocalise. A voice **prosthesis** can be implanted in the neck. The prosthesis produces a noise when the stoma is covered, and the person breathes out through the implanted valve.

The valve produces a noise which can be used to makes words by moving the mouth and lips in the usual way to allow for speech. For those with tracheostomies, it is possible for the patient to produce sounds that can be identifiable speech. The cuff on the tracheostomy tube can be deflated, or a tube with no cuff can be inserted. This works by allowing the air of the exhaled breath to bypass the tube and be redirected to the larynx to produce sounds (Hess, 2005). There are additional options of using a one-way speaking valve on the tracheostomy tube to increase **phonation**. Less commonly, the patient could use a clean finger to obstruct or occlude the tracheostomy tube, opening on exhalation, redirecting the breath to produce sounds.

It is also possible to use the **oesophagus** for speech, which is a technique where the person pushes air through the oesophagus. As the air moves along, it vibrates and makes a noise which can be manipulated to produce words using the lips and mouth.

The external means of generating sounds for speech for a laryngectomy is via the electrolarynx, which is a small battery-operated device that vibrates to produce sound when it is held under the chin. The electrical vibrations pick up the movement of the mouth and lips which can be translated into speech.

Principles of inclusive communication

When communicating with a group or a community, we need to presume that there are people within those groups with a range of needs and differences when it comes to communication.

As we touched on in Chapter 6, communication that is inclusive of those differences and needs should be considered at all times. Good practice in communication that is inclusive allows you to reach the target audience in a more effective and efficient way and allows people to access services equally. Understanding all of the support mechanisms available to support communication that have been discussed in this chapter is essential. We will explore inclusive access to services in Activity 7.3.

Activity 7.3   Case study

You have been asked to be involved in the setting-up of a vaccination centre for a new vaccine targeting 60–70-year-old males. The trust has set up two temporary buildings in the car park at the rear of the hospital. One of the buildings will be for staff to consult with the patients about the vaccination; it has a joining door to the other building where the patients will receive the vaccination and where the vaccine is stored.

The vaccination is a one-dose vaccine, but this needs to be followed up by a blood test for antigens in six weeks' time. What measures do you think you should include for this service to be inclusive?

Sample answer to the question is provided at the end of the chapter.

Remember that communication is a two-way process, and it is important for the service user to feel heard and understood. If someone has a particular communication need that requires additional assistance, there must be sufficient time for the communication to take place. Booking a double appointment for someone who needs more time is a simple and effective way of supporting them.

Considering accessibility is also a key factor in effective communication, and making reasonable adjustments for different needs welcomes inclusion. Make sure signage is clear, in simple fonts and of an adequate size to be easily read. You may want to include braille, have large-print leaflets, letters and appointment cards. Keep areas well lit and uncluttered, have induction loops for hearing aid users and automatically opening doors for those who use mobility aids, carers and service animals.

Staff training is essential to ensure they acquire the skills of delivering nonjudgemental communication and having patience. Staff should be able to effectively assess whether someone needs additional support with communication. They should know how to access that support, how to use devices and how to alter their behaviour to flexibly maximise inclusive communication.

Finally, involve the users of the service to gauge their opinion and needs when seeking to improve inclusivity. Adding a translation service may be at an additional cost, but if it is effective and encourages positive health changes and increased user satisfaction, then the cost can be justified (Scottish Government, 2011).

Chapter summary

This chapter has considered what a sensory impairment is and has explored other aspects that can influence effective communication. It has introduced some of the supportive tools to aid communication with people experiencing difficulties and how we can be inclusive of those difficulties when delivering health services.

Activities: Brief outline answers

Activity 7.1 Work-based learning (page 121)

Question 1:

Starting with 'Hello, my name is' and your name, you would greet Brandon with 'They Kennedy, can I call you Brandon?'

Make the pronoun prominent on the documentation for Brandon and ensure this is handed over to all staff in the day care unit for the day to ensure no offence is caused.

Take the time to make sure Brandon understands what is going to happen and allow time for questions.

While Brandon is in the department, they should be allowed the communication aids, the magazines and their glasses on as long as possible before needing to be transferred to the theatre, and all items should be returned to Brandon as soon as possible on leaving theatre.

Brandon should be placed out of a draft and with sufficient blankets to keep them warm. Brandon should have access to a nurse call bell in easy reach.

Brandon states that they would like to see what is going on in the department. This might not be appropriate for they to see other patients, but in order for Brandon not to feel isolated, they should be placed near to the nurses' station so they can see activity.

Question 2. Some of the images might be:

A pain assessment chart with facial images, which express stages of pain on a scale of 1 (being no pain) to 10 (being intense pain).

A glass of water to indicate whether he is thirsty (being mindful to give Brandon advice on not rinsing their mouth, to avoid dry socket after the teeth had been removed).

A picture of a mobile phone to indicate that Brandon would like to text/get you to speak to Jackie.

A picture of a toilet. An image of a blanket to assess whether Brandon is cold. Other images could include pictures which indicate whether it is too loud, good, bad, stop. There may also be images on who, where, when, what.

This is not an exhaustive list.

Activity 7.2 Work-based learning: braille and visual impairment (see the answers to the braille examples in Figures 12-7, 7.14, 7.15, 7.16 and 7.17) (page 128)

1.
Figure 7.12
Answer: Hello my name is Anne.
2.
Figure 7.14
Answer: Take 75mgs of Aspirin one a day.
3.
Figure 7.15
Answer: 42
4.
Figure 7.16
Answer: 9330
5.
Figure 7.17
Answer: NHS

Activity 7.3 Case study (page 131)

Accessibility: make sure the service is clearly signposted from the front of the hospital and along the route to the vaccination centre. Making the signage in a large simple font that makes it easy to read with a braille option is ideal.

Will you need a ramp to get in and out of the buildings, or do you need a handrail? There is likely to be some mobility issues with this population section. So, making sure the doors will accommodate a wheelchair is good and allowing people to be able to sit while they wait is considerate to their needs. The seating should be robust and of an adequate height, which enables a person to sit and rise with minimal assistance.

Making sure the area is well lit and uncluttered reduces the trips and falls risk.

Staff training: staff need to be able to assess whether someone requires additional support with their communication and if they need more time for the consultation. A non-judgemental and patient approach is essential.

Supportive devices: consider, does the person need the information in large print or in braille, do they use an augmented communication device or need the use of the loop induction system for hearing-aid users? It might mean they need a translator, an advocate, or responsible person to assist them. Consider the use of an inclusive call system, which verbally calls for the patients, as well as using text.

This is not an exhaustive answer.

Knowledge review

Now that you have worked through this chapter, how would you rate your knowledge of the following topics?

	Good	Adequate	Poor
• the definition of 'sensory impairment'			
• the use of alternative communications tools which are age appropriate			
• the use of alternative communications tools which are cognitively appropriate			
• the use and application of braille, BSL and Makaton			
• inclusive communication			

If you are unsure of some aspects, what are you going to do next?

Further reading and useful websites

For more information on the development of art from artists using their feet or mouth:
www.mfpa.uk/about-mfpa/who-we-are

For more information and links to further activities and resources for those with hearing impairments, visit the Royal National Institute for Deaf people (RIND): **https://rnid.org.uk/**

Explore more content and activities involving BSL: **www.british-sign.co.uk/**

For more information and links to further activities for the sight impaired, visit the Royal National Institute of Blind People (RNIB) webpages: **www.rnib.org.uk/?gclid=EAIaIQobChMIoNOUrcO_8gIVje3tCh0rdwzoEAAY ASAAEgIK3PD_BwE**

Tinnitus association: **www.tinnitus.org.uk/blog/more-people-living-with-tinnitus-than-previously-thought**

For more information on the communication passport and some templates, please visit the Communication Matters webpage: **www.communicationmatters.org.uk/what-is-aac/types-of-aac/communication-passports/**

For more information on the hypersensitivity and sensory overload that can affect a person with an autism spectrum disorder, please visit the National Autistic society at: **www.autism.org.uk/**

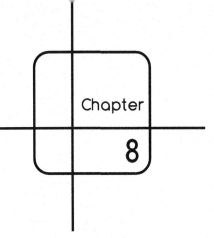

Chapter

8

Assessment and support in clinical practice for the nursing associate role

Demonstrate effective skills when working in teams through:

4.1   active listening when receiving feedback and when dealing with team members' concerns and anxieties.

5.   Demonstrate effective supervision skills by providing:

5.1   clear instructions and explanations when supervising others.

5.2   clear instructions and checking understanding when delegating care responsibilities to others.

5.3   clear constructive feedback in relation to care delivered by others.

5.4   encouragement to colleagues that helps them to reflect on their practice.

Chapter aims

By the end of this chapter, you will be able to:

- understand what being a role model means.
- how to give positive feedback.
- understand the process of decision making.
- understand what shared decision making is.
- explore the use of patient decision aids (PDA).

Introduction

For those of us drawn to healthcare, the goal is to have a positive impact on the lives of those we care for; even in the darkest of times, we aim to shine a light and offer solace to help get people through the darkness. As we continue to focus on communication, this chapter will be building human capital by realising the impact and the potential of every nursing associate. As elements of clinical practice, knowledge and experience embed themselves in the working day of the nursing associate. Becoming a role model for others is a natural process. This chapter asks the reader to embark on a journey towards recognising their impact on others, becoming a supervisor and making effective decisions as a nursing associate moves towards leadership. This chapter will explore what a role model is and what skills are required. We then move on to making decisions.

Expectations in being a leader for training, and the nursing associate

When the NMC (2018c) developed the Nursing Associate Proficiencies, they also considered the platforms for practice for the nursing associate in comparison to the registered nurse. Figure 8.1 outlines the expectations of each of the roles, as well as the key differences and similarities within them.

Nursing Associate	Registered Nurse
1. Be an accountable professional 2. Promoting health and preventing ill health 3. Provide and monitor care 4. Working in teams 5. Improving safety and quality of care 6. Contributing to integrated care	1. Be an accountable professional 2. Promoting health and preventing ill health 3. Assessing needs and planning care 4. Providing and evaluating care 5. Leading and managing nursing care and working in teams 6. Improving safety and quality of care 7. Coordinating care

Figure 8.1   NMC platform for practice.

At first glance, it may appear that as a registered nursing associate, your role does not extend to assessing and supervising a student, but you would be wrong. The NMC recognises the value in you and the experience you have to assess and supervise new and emerging registered nurses and nursing associates. The role of the assessor and supervisors is not one to be feared, but to be embraced. Learning, like communication, is a two-way process when it is done right. Engaging on supervision helps you to understand more about yourself and develops you as a person and a nursing associate, as much as it helps and supports the new learning of a student.

Being a role model

The moment you register as a nursing associate, there becomes a responsibility to uphold the integrity of that qualification and, before you even think about being a supervisor, you are a role model first. You are the one that the students will look up to and will want to learn from. They want to get your approval that they are doing a good job. But what is that job and what does role modelling look like for nurses?

- Empathy: being able to understand the feelings of others.
- Emotionally stable or resilient: able to manage difficult emotions or situations that cause upset, and the ability to bounce back from them.
- Good communicator: one of the most important qualities of any healthcare professional. If communication fails, it can have dire consequences for people.
- Versatile/flexible: able to adapt to difference situations and activities. Willingness to work weekends and night duty.
- Physical stamina: the ability to endure long hours on your feet and work physically hard.

So, these are the common attributes to being a nurse, but what about other aspects of being a role model? In Activity 8.1, you can explore what other attributes a role model may have.

Activity 8.1   Reflection: role models

Think about a time when you were influenced by a role model. It can be from any part of your life and be from any aspect of your experience. Now ask yourself:

What made them a good role model?

List a few of the attributes that they had which made them someone you could look up to.

In Activity 8.1, you reflected on your role model and the factors that influenced you. Baldwin et al. (2014) as cited by Owen (2018) stated that good role models are approachable and instil confidence in others. They create an atmosphere that is easy and relaxed because they facilitate the learning and the development of others. Role models provide positive examples of how we should practise and behave.

When considering role modelling within nursing, we would do well to reflect on the 6Cs and the 4Ps (Chapter 3). Along with the desirable attributes identified in the two models, we need to go further to consider areas that are less quantifiable. Nurses can demonstrate compassion, competency and so on, but there are areas that are harder to define and cannot be taught. Being a good person is one such aspect. Having passion for the role, which gives someone the fire from inside to be able to be a strong advocate for patients and colleagues, is another, as well as the openness of spirit to be willing to share experiences, and the desire to learn (Truman, 2019).

What we do know is that positive role modelling is a good way to support learning in practice. A study from 2017 noted that it led to increased learner satisfaction from both university and in practice (Jack et al., 2017). So, knowing that having a role model has a positive effect on education, we know that as a registered nursing associate, there is an expectation that the role will include supervision and the assessment of others in training.

Being a supervisor or assessor and being a role model in leadership is less about being a good person and is more about being emotionally intelligent and reflective. A common phrase we think of when we think about leadership is 'to lead by example' (NHS Leadership Academy, 2013). What does this really mean? It is not about people blindly following in your footsteps; it is about showing others what is possible. You are guiding people with your behaviour and inspiring others.

Offering inspiration and outlining the possibilities is not all. A role model reflects commitment to the service and all patients and colleagues, which means hard work. An effective role model should be prepared to 'muck in' and get involved. If there is a bed that needs cleaning and making, clean and make it yourself and do it well. If a water jug needs filling, fill it. If lunches need giving out, give them out and do full bed baths. However, it is not possible to do it all and neither should you be expected to. Being a role model also involves leadership skills. This will enable you to identify the resources available and the appropriate delegation of tasks according to the workload, as well as the need and the skills of available personnel.

As linked to the NMC *Code* (2018a) point 20.8, being trusted and respected are essential aspects of being a good role model, but trust and respect are not automatic and are earned through a process of being fair, honest and consistent. Colleagues need to know that you have their best interests at heart and will support them, no matter what. Certainly, a role model must demonstrate integrity, not engage in behaviour that is unprofessional or distasteful and not tolerate those behaviours in others. A role model should show positivity and persistence in their behaviour. Nursing is unpredictable and can be very challenging and the ability to handle these situations with positivity and resolve pulls people together to get the job done. Lastly, and most importantly, a role model should be accountable and take responsibility for their actions. Everyone makes mistakes and the important thing for any healthcare professional to do is admit that mistake and own it. Do not blame others or make excuses, but take clear action to correct and report the situation (Bussard and Lawrence, 2019).

In Activity 8.2, there is an opportunity to explore your current attributes to being a good role model and supervisor and what you may need to develop further to meet the expectations of the NMC in becoming a supervisor and then an assessor in practice.

Activity 8.2 Reflection: skills to lead

Your line manager is really pleased with your development and wants you to think about taking on the role of being a supervisor for the next intake of nursing associate students.

Take a few minutes to think about how you currently engage in supporting others; these others could be patients and/or other staff and colleagues. Jot down a few points on each of the sections of this S.W.O.T. analysis. S.W.O.T. stands for strengths, weaknesses, opportunities and threats.

To get you started, there are a few suggestions added to each box and a brief explanation of areas to think about (see Figure 8.2). The question you should keep in mind during this activity is 'what does a supervisor need to do, and what can I do?'

	Strengths	Weaknesses
Internal	• Professional qualification and experience. • •	• Lack confidence in my knowledge. • •
	Opportunities	Threats
External	• There are new students starting soon. • •	• The ward is always really busy, and I don't want to get distracted. • •

Figure 8.2   S.W.O.T. analysis.

Some more possible/suggested answers to the S.W.O.T. can be found at the end of the chapter.

In Activity 8.2, you were able to explore strengths and weakness, opportunities and threats to developing yourself into a good role model as a supervisor and assessor.

As we have seen throughout the book, communication is central to relationships and effective care delivery. As part of the process of care delivery, there are many decisions that need to be made along the way.

Decision making

Various sources have tried to establish the number of decisions a person makes in a day. The general estimate is that your average adult will make 35,000 decisions during the course of a day. Decision making is an analytical and intuitive process; the analytical aspect combines information from the patient and knowledge from an evidence base, whereas the intuitive element comes from prior experience and learned responses and similarities (Nibblelink and Brewer, 2018). Decision making requires the ability to process complex information (Nibblelink and Brewer, 2018), which, in nursing, can be challenged by the lack of time, resources and information.

Activity 8.3   Decision making

You are stood exactly in the middle of 12-bedded day surgery recovery. On the list today has been Arthroscopy surgeries (knee joint investigations). All the beds are taken by people recovering from the same procedure. In the same moment, two call buzzers are activated by patients wanting assistance. Your colleagues are all busy, so it is up to you to decide which patient to attend to first. You notice one of the buzzers was from bed 1 and the other from bed 12. These beds are the same distance from you but are in the opposite direction of each other.

Which patient will you see to first? Bed 1 or bed 12?

Why did you make that decision?

How did you come to that decision?

Would any extra information have helped you make that decision? What else would you liked to have known?

Some suggested answers are discussed at the end of the chapter.

As we have seen in Activity 8.3, decisions aren't always easy and there aren't always clear options.

Making a decision uses the same process, no matter what that decision is (see Figure 8.3). We use the same decision-making process for setting an alarm, choosing dinner, or deciding the type of dressing to use on a leg wound and whether to start CPR.

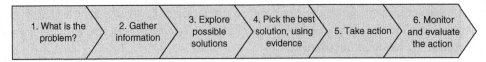

Figure 8.3 Decision-making process.

The best decisions in practice are made with a combination of current research evidence, own clinical experiences and understanding the needs and the preferences of the patient, regardless of the care setting (see Figure 8.3). However, there are challenges to decision making in healthcare because the speed in which decisions need to be made can vary dramatically. In emergency situations, the decisions are often very complex, involving many different factors for consideration, but these decisions need to be made quickly and in rapid succession. Where rapid decisions are expected this is referred to as an implied response time (Thompson et al., 2004). To aid decisions that need to be done quickly, a decision tree can be used. A decision tree is a visual algorithm that can be negotiated at a glance to advise on treatment options and the next steps based on clinical data (Dowding and Thompson, 2004). An example of the decision tree can be seen in the National Early Warning Score (NEWS) or NEWS2 (Royal College of Physicians, 2017) chart, but these can be used in any number of places and situations where clinical outcomes can be predicted.

Other factors include the availability of some resources. It could be that the latest research states that using dressing A is the perfect solution to the wound problem; however, dressing A is not recognised by the National Institute for Health and Clinical Excellence (NICE) and not available from the dressings formulary, so cannot be prescribed.

Reflecting on your experience, it will be evident that having time to make a decision is a luxury in healthcare. This is where the final element of the decision-making process becomes vital. The monitoring and evaluation of the actioned decision helps to assess how well something is working, or not (Moule et al., 2017). The process of evaluation is there to consider whether a patient has improved, and the actions were effective, or whether the patient is worse, experiencing a reaction or there is no improvement. In these last instances, the decision process starts again, starting with establishing what the problem is. It could be the same problem as before, or there could be a new or additional problem. During the process of evaluation, it may be necessary to repeat the assessment using the same decision tree and noting any differences, as you would do in a Waterlow score or a NEWS2. Repeating the assessment can bring valuable insight into the situation, much as doing base line observations can help monitor a person's responses to treatment or general health status. Regardless of the result of the evaluation, our main aim is to benefit the patient and get the best outcome for them, but what it does for the healthcare professional is to give more evidence, education and experience to help with future decisions.

Shared decision making

Shared decision making is the process within which the nursing associate works together with the person to reach a decision about their care (NICE, 2021a). These decisions take into account the evidence and the person's individual preferences, beliefs, values and culture.

The nursing associate role in this instance is to use information from the patient, your knowledge and evidence base, which includes research evidence and own experience to form an informed and mutually satisfactory decision (see Figure 8.4). Shared decision making is a collaboration between the patient and the healthcare professional. It could be about someone's immediate care needs or could be for a future event, such as with advance care planning.

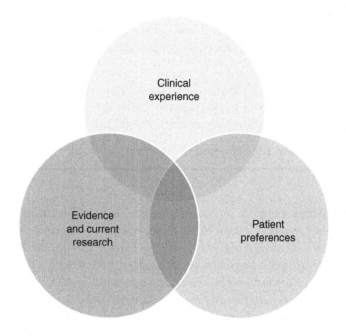

Figure 8.4 Shared decision making.

For the patient, they feel more informed on the decisions surrounding their care and they will understand the potential benefits and risks as a result of the action taken on that joint decision (NICE, 2021a). In Activity 8.4, we look at how to identify an opportunity for a health promotion intervention using shared decision making.

Activity 8.4   Shared decision making: work-based learning

In this activity, we will use imaginative role and work-based resources to explore shared decision making. Please refer to the further reading session at the end of the chapter and look up the copy of the smoking cessation PDA from York NHS Trust.

(Continued)

(Continued)

Scenario

Shauna is a 27-year-old woman who is being visited by you for a routine baby check. Baby India was born ten days ago at 39 weeks, weighing 5lbs/2.2kg. You note that baby India is underweight and appears to be a little nasally congested.

When you enter the home, you also noted cigarette smoke in the air, and you are concerned about baby India's exposure to second-hand smoke. Shauna confirms she smokes but that she has cut down since the baby was born. Shauna also confirmed she has smoked during her pregnancy and had tried to stop before, but it didn't work.

Consider this information and Shauna's previous desire and attempt to stop smoking, as well as using the PDA. How will you approach the topic of smoking cessation with Shauna? What kind of questions do you think you should ask?

Some suggested answers are discussed at the end of the chapter.

Activity 8.4 is a prime example of how to use the Health Education England (HEE) (2016) Make Every Contact Count (MECC) work. Being a nursing associate enables you to spend more time with a patient to truly understand what matters to them and what motivates their health behaviours. Working together with your patient leaves them feeling more informed on the decisions surrounding their care and they will understand the potential benefits and risks as a result of the action taken on that joint decision (NICE, 2021b). A patient also feels the interaction is more meaningful and empowering, and it is a more rewarding experience for the healthcare professionals (Pieterse et al., 2019).

As much as shared decision making sounds like the obvious, clear and practical approach to communication, however, there remain challenges. When it comes to consent and capacity of thought, we need the patient to fully understand what is being asked of them and what the medical procedures and treatments mean in real terms. Otherwise, it becomes confusing and anxiety-provoking for the patient.

The other crucial aspect to know is that patients cannot request treatment options which are not supported by the evidence. They can only refuse offers of treatment (dissent) (Mental Capacity Act: HMSO, 2005). A silly example of this would be as follows: a patient presents at A&E with a heavy nosebleed (epistaxis) that occurred spontaneously and has lasted for over one hour. A discussion with the patient reveals that they are refusing or dissenting to have nasal cautery (NICE, 2020), which is the standard evidence-based treatment for this condition. Instead, they are insisting that the proper treatment is to have their feet bandaged together and soaked in saline, and they are demanding this is done as soon as possible.

In this instance, we would try and educate the patient regarding the treatment options. We would not force a patient to have any treatment or procedure they did not consent to (if they are able to give consent), but equally we would not perform any procedure that has no evidence base or rationale, or one that was not lawful.

Chapter summary

This chapter has considered the development of the professional nursing associate towards becoming a positive role model for colleagues and supervisor and assessor for new learners, while maintaining a professional approach and behaviour. The chapter has also introduced activities that stretch the reader to explore intelligent decision making, collaborative communication in caring and using opportunities to go beyond task-orientated care and making every contact count.

Activities: Brief outline answers

Activity 8.2 Reflection: skills to lead (page 140)

	Strengths	Weaknesses
Internal	• Professional qualification and experience. • Hard working. • I understand exactly what they are going through. • Keen to support others with the opportunity to be a nursing associate.	• Lack confidence in my knowledge. • Time management and organisation. • I don't think they would take me seriously. • I don't know how to manage a problem student.
	Opportunities	Threats
External	• There are new students starting soon. • It would improve my confidence. • My line manager thinks I can do it. • I can reflect on when I was under supervision.	• The ward is always really busy, and I don't want to get distracted. • More experienced members of staff might judge me. • I don't know how to supervise someone. • If I get it wrong, will I lose my registration?

Figure 8.5 This is not an exhaustive list, and may not match with your S.W.O.T.

Activity 8.3 Decision making (page 141)

Which patient will you see to first? Bed 1 or bed 12?

Why did you make that decision?

How did you come to that decision?

Would any extra information have helped you make that decision? What else would you liked to have known?

This is an ethical dilemma that is based on consequences and the balance of reducing harm, which is firmly linked to professional accountability. In this instance, there is no right answer, but there is a consequence for one of the patients, in the fact they have to wait longer. The question is whether that is fair. The answer is ambiguous. It is not fair that someone must wait longer than another to be seen; however, it is fair because there was no judgement made against the one who had to wait. The treatment was equal, and we need to accept that someone will always have to wait.

So, what if you had more information, what would change?

What if bed 1 was a 60-year-old woman and bed 12 was a 26-year-old man. Whom would you choose?

We have some more information for you. Bed 1 was doing her third marathon when, in her last mile, she slipped and injured her knee, which lead to her procedure today. Bed 12 was in the process of escaping from the police when his injury occurred. He had to jump a wall, but being 20 stone in weight (280lbs/127kgs), he could not clear the wall and fell badly. Whom do you choose now?

None of this additional information should make any difference to your first decision, but this is where human nature gets brought into decision making. The additional information would have made you form a judgement, whether positive or negative, and most people will choose the most personally favourable option first. Being aware that there is a dilemma and that there will be consequences, while being able to reflect on your decisions and feelings, is key to being an emotionally intelligent decision maker.

Activity 8.4 Shared decision making: work-based learning (page 143)

As a shared decision, it is important to establish the reasons behind her health behaviours and give her information of the effects on her health and the health of the baby as a means of supporting Shauna's decision process.

Questioning to establish her understanding may include: (not necessarily in this order)

Did she realise that smoking around a baby can be the cause of an increased risk of sudden infant death syndrome?

It can also cause you and the baby pneumonia and other breathing issues.

Why do you think you smoke? How long have you been smoking for? What health implications are there for Shauna which you could explore?

Do you have any concerns about stopping smoking? Such as gaining weight. Particularly after just having a baby, weight may be a factor in staying as a smoker.

Do you think there are any obstacles to stopping smoking? (Such as does your partner/family smoke?)

What is it about smoking you enjoy? Here you can explore different treatment options. Explore the cost of smoking.

These questions are trying to establish the basis of Shauna's health behaviours and choices. According to the Health Belief model (Becker, 1974), people will not change their behaviour unless they can perceive themselves to be at risk, or, in this example, in the instance that the baby India is at risk. To challenge health beliefs, it is important to allow Shauna to explore the pros and cons of smoking versus stopping smoking and what she would consider to be acceptable as a form of treatment or help. More information on the Health Belief model can be found in the further reading section at the end of the chapter.

One of the most important aspects for discussion when exploring a change in health behaviour is to be non-judgemental and to explain it is okay to fail when making a health behaviour change, as each failure is an opportunity to learn about the triggers which pre-empted the failure. The point is that they learn from the 'failures' and try again. More information on this can be found in the further reading section at the end of the chapter under the transformational theories of behaviour change model.

Knowledge review

Now that you have worked through this chapter, how would you rate your knowledge of the following topics?

	Good	Adequate	Poor
• being a role model			
• positive feedback			
• the process of decision making			
• shared decision making			
• the use of PDAs			

If you are unsure of some aspects, what are you going to do next?

Further reading and useful websites

Standards from NICE on the PDAs:
www.nice.org.uk/corporate/ecd8

More information on the transformational theories of behaviour change model:
https://pubmed.ncbi.nlm.nih.gov/10170434/#:~:text=The%20transtheoretical %20model%20posits%20that,action%2C%20maintenance%2C%20and%20 termination

More information on the Health Belief model:
https://study.com/academy/lesson/health-belief-model-in-nursing-definition-theory-examples.html#:~:text=Health%20Belief%20Model%20 as%20Nursing,behavior%20to%20prevent%20the%20problem

An example of a PDA produced by NICE for the treatment of high blood pressure: **www.nice.org.uk/guidance/ng136/resources/how-do-i-control-my-blood-pressure-lifestyle-options-and-choice-of-medicines-patient-decision-aid-pdf-6899918221**

Read more about the HEE MECC work and the impact it could have on public health and health behaviours: **www.england.nhs.uk/wp-content/uploads/2016/04/making-every-contact-count.pdf**

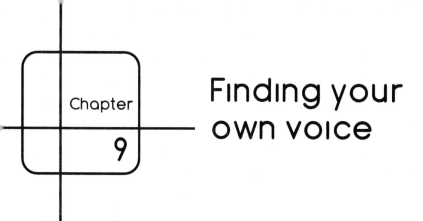

Finding your own voice

NMC FUTURE NURSE STANDARDS OF PROFICIENCY FOR NURSING ASSOCIATES

This chapter will address the following platforms and proficiencies:

Platform 1: Being an accountable professional

At the point of registration, the nursing associate will be able to:

1.15 take responsibility for continuous self-reflection, seeking and responding to support and feedback to develop professional knowledge and skills.

1.16 act as an ambassador for their profession and promote public confidence in health and care services.

Platform 3: Provide and monitor care

At the point of registration, the nursing associate will be able to:

3.24 take personal responsibility to ensure that relevant information is shared according to local policy and appropriate immediate action is taken to provide adequate safeguarding and that concerns are escalated.

Platform 4: Working in teams

At the point of registration, the nursing associate will be able to:

4.1 demonstrate an awareness of the roles, responsibilities and scope of practice of different members of the nursing and interdisciplinary team, and their own role within it.

4.2 demonstrate an ability to support and motivate other members of the care team and interact confidently with them.

(Continued)

(Continued)

Platform 5: Improving safety and quality of care

At the point of registration, the nursing associate will be able to:

5.10 understand their own role and the roles of all other staff at different levels of experience and seniority in the event of a major incident.

Annexe A: Communication and relationship management skills

At the point of registration, the nursing associate will be able to safely demonstrate the following skills:

4. Communication skills for working in professional teams:

Demonstrate effective skills when working in teams through:

4.1 active listening when receiving feedback and when dealing with team members' concerns and anxieties.

4.3 being a calm presence when exposed to situations involving conflict.

4.4 being assertive when required.

Chapter aims

By the end of this chapter, you will be able to:

- explore the types of leadership styles.
- consider your leadership style.
- understand the skill of delegation.
- explore how to assess competency.
- find your voice within the team.

Introduction

As we have seen in the previous chapter, as a nursing associate, you are not required to lead on and manage care decisions and the clinical environment; however, you are required to lead within a team when working with others and the multidisciplinary team. Within this chapter, we will be exploring leadership and management styles and developing your leadership voice.

The first aspect of developing that leadership voice and communicating as a leader is understanding the different styles and types of leadership. In this next section, we will explore some of the more commonly known leadership styles.

Autocratic/authoritarian leadership

Autocratic or authoritarian leadership is when an individual is in control of all decisions. This style of leader will make decisions based on their own ideas, experiences and judgements without the advice from others.

Their approach is 'I know best' and they require absolute control over a group. There is often a very clear separation between the leader and the group to be led. If you can imagine a drill sergeant in the US Army, or the equivalent Warrant Officer role in the British Army, this would be the ultimate example of an autocratic leader.

In terms of communication, in general, the autocratic leader does not need to shout like a drill sergeant, although in a loud setting, it might be required.

There are definite pros and cons to the autocratic style of leadership. In emergency situations, having one person take charge and make the decisions quickly and effectively is preferable because it allows others to focus on their roles without needing to make complex decisions, and it gives a clear chain of command.

Outside of urgent and stressful situations, the autocratic style can limit creativity, stifles the group's contribution and limits team growth. This ultimately damages team morale and can cause resentment when the leader is seen as bossy, controlling or like a dictator.

Charismatic/visionary leadership

'Charisma' comes from the Greek for 'grace' or 'gift'. The 'gift' is being a very skilled and eloquent communicator who can communicate on a deep, emotional level. They can express a compelling and captivating vision and are able to persuade and motivate others by stimulating emotion and passion in them. As much as this leadership style creates positivity in the role, it relies heavily on the leader to make the decisions and does not allow for others to grow and develop.

Bureaucratic leadership

Bureaucratic leadership is in contrast to charismatic leadership, in the fact that it is impersonal and focused on the needs of the organisation, not the individual. It has a clearly defined chain of command. Bureaucratic leaders prefer to follow rules and regulations which favour getting predictable outcomes.

Bureaucratic leadership is an interesting concept when it comes to healthcare service provision. Bureaucracy is more associated with public sector work, such as local government and areas which use public money or taxation. The health service falls into that category in terms of funding, and the service is very hierarchical; where it fails is in predictability. Activity 9.1 will explore bureaucratic leadership in healthcare provision.

Activity 9.1   Work-based learning: meeting targets

You are a nursing associate working in primary care in a GP surgery. You have been asked to review the data relevant to the uptake of cervical smears within the practice, to

(Continued)

(Continued)

ensure the surgery meets the Quality Outcome Framework (QOF) indicators for funding. Specifically, indicator CS005 (BMA, 2020). QOF is a voluntary programme directed towards GP services in England; its aim is to standardise the delivery of care within primary care. The QOF, as a government initiative, offers GPs a financial incentive to meet national targets in identifying and monitoring chronic conditions, such as diabetes and asthma. It also has a focus on monitoring reducing risk factors associated with developing cancer.

Indicator ID CS005 is the QOF looking at cervical screening

The proportion of women eligible for screening and aged 25–49 years at the end of period reported whose notes record that an adequate cervical screening test has been performed in the previous three years and six months.

Points allocation: 14 (each point is worth £194.83).

Payment thresholds: 45–80%.

Points accrued for lower performance threshold (under 45%): 3.

So what numbers are we looking at?

How many women are there estimated to be in England?

a. 34,761,863
b. 12,673,089
c. 23,495,116

How many women between 29 years and 49 years old are there estimated to be in England?

a. 3,476,999
b. 2,338,147
c. 1,024,699

What is the average size of a GP surgery in England?

a. 3,167
b. 1,980
c. 2,087

What is the estimated percentage of women aged 25 to 49 years old who are registered with a GP in England?

a. 5.2%
b. 3.9%
c. 2.9%

What is the percentage national uptake of cervical smears in England?

a. 36.5%
b. 61.8%
c. 72.2%

(NHS Digital, 2020)

Work out the average number of women aged 25 years to 49 years who are regis-tered with the average size GP in England.

a.   60 patients
b.   53 patients
c.   81 patients

Working based on the average percentage number of smears done according to the national uptake in England data, how many patients would the average GP surgery expect to attend for cervical smears?

a.   65 patients
b.   43 patients
c.   52 patients

If 1 QOF point equals £194.83 and you had the national average number of patients attending the average surgery for their smears, how much could the GP surgery earn for that QOF target being met (considering the points are 14 per person)?

a.   £117,287.66
b.   £87,451.78
c.   £231,655.98

If the average surgery had only 22% of their 25–49-year-old female patients attend their cervical smear, how much would the surgery earn in QOF points (considering the points reduce to three per patient)?

a.   £65,981.01
b.   £10,443.12
c.   £7,598.37

What would be the financial difference between a high-performing and low-performing average GP?

a.   £109,689.29
b.   £77,008.66
c.   £165,674.92

Answers are available at the end of the chapter.

As we can see in Activity 9.1, bureaucratic leadership focuses on targets and money rather than people and experiences. The government sets the QOF indicators and the regulations on how to meet the standard, as well as the financial rewards for meeting those standards. The GP service then relies on predictable factors of a disease to target; for example, all women between 29 and 49 for a cervical smear. The key here is that they are targeting age and gender and not the women directly who meet the criteria for testing; the human consideration is a secondary component to meeting the standard.

We know that people as personalities are not necessarily predictable, and it can lead to significant challenges to healthcare delivery. So focusing on hard targets can be easier, if not always appropriate for all situations and scenarios.

Laissez-faire leadership

Laissez-faire leadership is a style which relies heavily on delegation to others and minimal participation in decision making or the giving of direction. This style of leadership encourages the employees to take the lead in decision making and to solve their own problems, which works well with an experienced and knowledgeable team. This style is good for the personal development of the employee, but the lack of direction can lead to job insecurity and anxiety among the staff. Glambek et al. (2017) make the link to job insecurity and workplace bullying. The lack of robust leadership was also a factor which led to workplace bullying in the Mid Staffordshire NHS Trust failing, as identified in the Francis Report (2013).

Democratic/participative leadership

Democratic or participative leadership has an identified leader. That leader works with the individuals in the group to work together to engage with the process of making a decision. It values individual ideas and encourages discussion and creativity. This style of leadership generates the highest productivity and boosts morale because the participants in the decision have a degree of ownership for the decision.

The success of this form of leadership does rely on the groups being experienced and knowledgeable, and it may lead to conflict if managed poorly or if the concept under discussion is not outlined sufficiently at the start of the decision-making process.

Transformational leadership

Transformational leadership has some roots in the charismatic/visionary style of leadership in so much as it evokes emotion in the group, stimulates creativity and can focus on the skills of individuals within a group. Where the styles differ is in the position of the leader, which in this style is more akin to democratic or participative leadership and is where the leader works alongside the group to form a conclusion or generate a solution. This closeness between the leader and the group promotes respect and mutual growth and sets the transformational leader as a natural role model (Allen et al., 2016).

Transactional leadership

Transactional leaders share some similarities with the autocratic style of leadership, where targets and tasks are the aim and the role of those below the leader is to obey instructions. A transactional leader will monitor the performance of their staff closely to ensure expectations of their performance are met. These performances will be met with either a reward for work well done or a punishment if the performance is seen as poor.

There is a clear place for periods of transactional leadership in healthcare, such as during emergency situations, but a long-term approach could lead to resentment and frustration due to the lack of growth and development opportunities and the stifling of creativity in the workplace.

No one person fits 100% into one specific leadership style, particularly in healthcare. We have already seen that healthcare can be unpredictable and dynamic in its changing pace. These changes and challenges require healthcare leaders to adapt their leadership style in accordance with the situation and the challenges they face. In Activity 9.2, there will be an opportunity to explore what type of leadership style you adopt.

Activity 9.2   Leadership and management style

Having read about the different types of leadership styles, let's explore your strengths and weaknesses as a leader and look at how you may take part in leading in this short quiz.

There are five questions below. Read each one and choose the answer you think is most like you or what you would expect from a leader.

1. When a decision needs to be made, do you?

    a. Make the decision yourself and present the plan to the team with clear direction.
    b. Make others aware of the problem, so you will wait to see what solution they come up with.
    c. Make the final decision but encourage input from the team.
    d. Let individuals in the team find own solutions that work best for them.
    e. Work out if this is a new problem or whether someone else has already got a solution you can use.

2. How do you want the people in the team to feel?

    a. That they are well liked by me and that I understand them on an emotional level.
    b. That they have very clearly defined roles and responsibilities, with clear tasks to perform.
    c. That they are aware of the expectations of the role and the regulations to adhere to.
    d. Like they are in control.
    e. That they feel part of something which they can contribute to.

3. How would you best motivate people in the team?

    a. People should motivate themselves.
    b. People are motivated by emotions to improve and to do good.

(Continued)

(Continued)

    c. People are motivated when they feel included and valued.

    d. People are motivated by rewards and punishments.

    e. People are motivated by their performance being monitored.

3. If a member of the team makes a mistake, what do you think should happen?

    a. They should be reprimanded and punished.

    b. They should be able to sort out the mistake themselves.

    c. They need to have their performance closely monitored.

    d. They need some supportive feedback and some further guidance or training.

    e. They need to understand how disappointed everyone else is in them.

4. In your view, leaders perform best when...?

    a. They are left alone to get on with the decisions; they are the most experienced, after all.

    b. They give clear orders and directions to the team.

    c. They leave the staff alone to do their own thing.

    d. They ask for input from other people in the team.

    e. They work with the others in the team.

Analysis of your answers can be found at the end of the chapter.

Reflect on the outcome of the short quiz and your S.W.O.T. analysis from Activity 8.2 in Chapter 8, where you looked at being a supervisor and assessor. In Activity 9.3, re-look at the S.W.O.T. with the outcome of the Activity 9.2 quiz in mind and with reference to communication when using those leadership styles. Noting your leadership preferences is important. However, being aware of the other styles allows you to be an adaptable leader. In Activity 9.1, we saw the need for a bureaucratic method when looking at data and hard facts; now, this same leadership style would not work if you were discussing how someone is feeling.

Activity: 9.3   Reflection on skills development

As much as leadership is not a defined role, as a nursing associate in management teams, you will still need to take on leadership qualities and make decisions.

Taking the next step from supervisor/assessor to leadership is a logical step in the development of the nursing associate role in practice.

Consider the answers you received from the short quiz and complete a reflective S.W.O.T. (see Figure 9.1) analysis on what you found out. What was good about what you found out, and are there any aspects you think you may need to change? What other methods might you use to find that leadership voice?

	Strengths	Weaknesses
Internal		
	Opportunities	Threats
External		

Figure 9.1 S.W.O.T. analysis.

This activity is subjective, so no model answers are supplied.

In Activity 9.3, we can clearly see the need for, and the value of, self-reflection in developing personally and professionally as it is an essential skill in all forms of healthcare delivery. However, as we know, we cannot deliver healthcare in isolation, and we need a team to perform efficiently and effectively in the provision of care. As a nursing associate, part of the healthcare team considering leadership style and awareness, the methods of communication within those styles becomes a vital part of the role when it comes to delegation.

Delegation

Delegation is defined by the NMC (2018b) as the transfer of a task or action to a competent individual who has the authority to perform the specific task in a specified situation.

The American Nurses Association and the National Council of State Boards of Nursing, as cited by Barrow and Sharma (2021), state that delegation is the process for a nurse to direct another person to perform nursing tasks and activities.

Delegation activities can occur between:

- at least one registered professional and another registered professional, or group of restraints;
- at least one registered professional to an unregulated member of the team, or group;
- at least one registered professional or unregistered team member to a carer(s) or family member(s).

(NMC, 2018b)

One of the interesting aspects of delegation is the principle of accountability and who has accountability when tasks are delegated. As we have seen, delegation involves at least two people: the 'delegator(s)', who offers or presents the task to be done, and the 'delegate(s)', who is the person who agrees to take on or accept the task as theirs to do (Barrow and Sharma, 2021).

The NMC (2018b) say that 'Accountability is the principle that individuals and organisations are responsible for their actions and may be required to explain them to others.'

With respect to delegation, all registered professionals, inclusive of registered nursing associates, are accountable for all aspects of their practice and retain accountability for what they choose to delegate to someone else. They take on accountability for tasks that are delegated to them and agreed upon. This is where choosing the right person for the right task at the right time and how to communicate the task becomes very important.

When you are delegating a task (NMC, 2018b)

It is the responsibility of the delegator(s) to make sure that:

- delegation does not harm the interests of people in your care. This means that you need to make sure that the team member(s) delegated to a task is fit to undertake it safely and with due respect to the patient and their current health status, situation or wishes and needs. For example, if there is a resident who needs personal care from two carers, due to mobility issues, but it is recorded in the patient notes that no males should attend to her personal care, then work should be allocated to ensure that two females can be available for the personal care of that resident.
- the task is within the other person's scope of competence. You must *know* that the team member(s) you are delegating to have the right level of experience and training to undertake the task safely. If the staff member(s) say they have the skills, you need to be certain. For example, if you need to take blood from someone and the person you delegate to says they have the venepuncture certificate, then you can be certain of their competence. If it then appears that they don't have that certificate and have not done the appropriate training, you remain accountable and responsible for the delegation and any injury that could have been caused to the patient(s) from that delegation. The person taking the blood and lying about their certification is also accountable for the harm caused, but, as the delegator, you retain the ultimate accountability.
- the person you are delegating to understands the boundaries of their own competence (see Figure 9.1). Do not mistake keenness for competence. Just because someone really wants to help, and they have seen an ECG a few times, does not mean that they are able to do that task. In these situations, it is important to remind the team member(s) of the boundaries. Similarly, people with limited knowledge cannot recognise the limits of their knowledge or intellect, and as such make poor choices based on the illusion of superiority

(Dunning and Kruger, 1999). As a person delegating, it is essential to recognise and manage the balance of actual competency against the inflated ego and incompetence of a team member(s).

- the person you are delegating to understands the task. This sounds like an obvious one, but what some people will nod and agree with may not be what you wanted them to do. Thinking back to Chapter 2, there are many drugs and treatments which share similar-sounding names. If what is being delegated is asking someone to do TPR (temperature, pulse and respirations) and they hear TPN (total parental nutrition), these are very different things. With accountability in mind, it is essential that understanding of the task is checked and confirmed.
- the person you are delegating to is clear about the circumstances in which they must refer to you. This is where clear communication in the delegation of a task is vital and in choosing the right words when delegating. For example, if you had an elderly patient who had been incontinent of urine and you need to delegate the changing of the bed to a team member(s), saying 'Can you please change Mrs Mallinson's bed?' is too vague. Do you mean changing the entire bed for another bed? Do you mean you want her changed to another bed space?

You could try: 'Mrs Mallinson has been incontinent, can you change her bed sheets, please?' Does this mean just the sheets? You would expect the pad and any bed clothes would be changed too. Although, this is not very patient centred.

So, you could try: 'Mrs Mallinson has been incontinent of urine. Can you make her comfortable with clean sheets, pads and night clothes please? And make sure you clean and review her skin. Report the condition of her skin to me once you have finished and let me know if there any specific changes noted.' 'I will check the notes to see if urinary incontinence is a new issue for Mrs Mallinson and whether we need to get a sample of urine.'

- you take reasonable steps to identify any risks and whether any supervision might be necessary. It is good practice in general to end any given set of instructions by saying 'let me know if you need any help or if you have a problem.' Although, if a known potential risk exists, then this must be factored into the planning of the task. For example, if you have a junior member of the team who is deemed competent in a task but lacks confidence in their ability, then supervision or guidance in this situation is prudent for the patient and would be supportive and developmental for the junior team member (see Figure 9.2).
- you take reasonable steps to monitor the outcome of the delegated task. Wherever possible, all delegated tasks should be followed up by the delegator, no matter how small. Even if this is a verbal check with the team member(s) to confirm if the free bad space has been cleaned and is ready for an admission, for example. Anything involving drugs/treatments/pain/comfort should be checked in person and documentation monitored. However, some tasks need to be delegated to a different shift, location or service, and, in these instances, checking on the outcomes is more difficult, which is where good written communication remains a key skill to effective, efficient and safe care delivery.

Dunning-Kruger effect

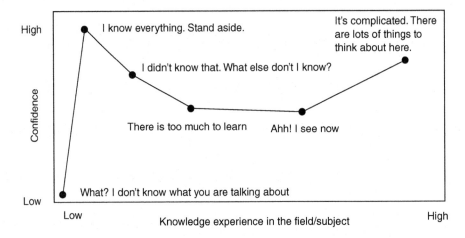

Figure 9.2 Based on the work by Dunning and Kruger. The Dunning-Kruger Effect (1999).

Chapter summary

Having a leadership voice is not about having a vast range of volume at your disposal or the means to project your voice. Effective leadership is not about being the biggest, boldest and most confident person in the room. Understanding yourself is a major factor in being an effective leader and recognising your style of leadership as a tool that you can use and which you can change. It is your choice. The ability to see past the person in front of you and what they portray, using your nursing skills of empathy, compassion and caring, can bring teams together and can make your voice the one worth listening to.

Activities: Brief outline answers

Activity 9.1 Work-based learning: meeting targets (page 151)

How many women are there estimated to be in England?

a. **34,761,863**
b. 12,673,089
c. 23,495,116

How many women between 29 years and 49 years old are there estimated to be in England?

a. 3,476,999
b. 2,338,147
c. **1,024,699**

What is the average size of a GP surgery in England?

a. 3,167
b. 1,980
c. **2,087**

What is the estimated percentage of women aged 25 to 49 years old who are registered with a GP in England?

a. 5.2%
b. 3.9%
c. **2.9%**

What is the percentage national uptake of cervical smears in England?

a. 36.5%
b. 61.8%
c. **72.2%**

(NHS Digital, 2020)

Work out the average number of women aged 25 to 49 who are registered with the average size GP in England.

a. **60 patients**
b. 53 patients
c. 81 patients

Working based on the average percentage number of smears done according to the national uptake in England data, how many patients would the average GP surgery be expecting to attend for cervical smears?

a. 65 patients
b. **43 patients**
c. 52 patients

If 1 QOF point equals £194.83 and you had the national average number patients attending the average surgery for their smears, how much could the GP surgery earn for that QOF target being met (considering the points are 14 per person)?

a. **£117,287.66**
b. £87,451.78
c. £231,655.98

If the average surgery had only 22% of their 25–49-year-old female patients attend their cervical smear, how much would the surgery earn in QOF points (considering the points reduce to three per patient)?

a. £65,981.01
b. £10,443.12
c. **£7,598.37**

What would be the financial difference between a high-performing and low-performing average GP?

a. **£109,689.29**
b. £77,008.66
c. £165,674.92

Activity 9.2 Leadership and management style (page 155)

Answers 1a, 2b, 3d, 4a and 5b are examples of autocratic leadership in practice, with 3d being a transactional example, which, as we have seen, has some roots in the autocratic style.

Answers 1b, 2a, 3b, 4e and 5e demonstrate charismatic leadership styles, with 3b and 5a including transformational traits.

Answers 1c, 2e, 3c, 4d, 5d indicate a democratic style of leadership.

Answers 1d, 2d, 3a, 4b, 5c are laissez-faire aspects of leadership.

Answers 1e, 2c, 3e, 4c, 5a are all examples of bureaucratic leadership.

Knowledge check

Now that you have worked through this chapter, how would you rate your knowledge of the following topics?

	Good	Adequate	Poor
• the types of leadership styles			
• your leadership style			
• the skill of delegation			
• how to assess competency			
• your voice within the team			

If you are unsure of some aspect, what are you going to do next?

Further reading and useful websites

For more information on leadership in healthcare:
www.kingsfund.org.uk/publications/leadership-and-leadership-development-health-care

Have you ever wondered about leadership styles? In this activity, you will find out which style you use:
www.leadershipacademy.nhs.uk/resources/healthcare-leadership-model/supporting-tools-resources/healthcare-leadership-model-self-assessment-tool/

For more information on the NMC's stance on delegation, visit the NMC online for more details:
www.nmc.org.uk/standards/code/code-in-action/delegation/

Glossary

acronym   a word or name that is formed from the initials or other aspects of a longer name or phrase. An example of an acronym can be found in the term NICE. NICE is the acronym for the National Institute of Clinical Excellence.

anterior   in medical terms, means facing to the 'front'.

apathy   a general lack of interest, sympathy, enthusiasm or concern. A synonym would be indifference.

asphyxia   a medical condition where someone is deprived of oxygen, often as a result of some form of suffocation. This can lead to the person becoming unconscious or death.

bilateral   it literary means 'both sides'. In medical terms, this can refer to organs, limbs or the right and left aspects of the body. For example, if someone had broken both ankles in an accident, this would be referred to as a bilateral fracture of the ankles.

candour   being truthful, open and honest.

fight or flight response   an automatic physiological reaction to an event that is seen as stressful or frightening. The prospect of a threat activates the sympathetic nervous system and triggers the body to respond to either fight or flee (Lamotte et al., 2021).

haptics   a system of non-verbal communication that uses touch or physical contact to convey language.

homeostatic   a state of balance or equilibrium in the body system(s), which works to maintain stability of the body functions to maintain health and for survival. The system is a self-regulating process which uses hormones and chemicals to balance bodily functions such as temperature and blood pressure.

hysterectomy   a surgical procedure to remove all or part of the uterus.

kinaesthesia   the process of the person being aware of the position and movement of parts of their body. This uses sensory organs in the muscles and joints to locate the actions and location of the body.

macroexpression   an extremely brief involuntary facial expression, which lasts between 0.5 to 4 seconds and is a true expression of personal feelings.

macular degeneration a degenerative condition, often associated with older age, which affects the central part of the back of the eye (the retina, the organ in the eye that senses light). The condition causes visual distortion and central vision loss.

microexpression a brief facial expression as the result of an emotional reaction to a stimuli/trigger. This expression quickly disappears when the individual wishes to conceal their true emotions in favour of a false emotional reaction.

mutism the inability to speak. This is usually because of deafness since birth or damage to the brain. It is also an unwillingness or refusal to speak that can be selective, which comes from a psychological cause, depression, trauma or as a coping mechanism.

oesophagus the muscular food pipe that connects the throat to the stomach.

oophorectomy a surgical procedure to remove one or both of the ovaries. The ovaries are small egg-shaped organs that sit on either side of the uterus. The ovaries are responsible for producing the hormones for a menstrual cycle and for producing the egg.

phonation the process of making speech sounds by the vibration of the vocal cords and vocal folds.

prosthesis in medicine, an artificial device that replaces either a missing or dysfunctioning part of the body. A prothesis is aimed at restoring the normal functions of the part being replaced.

proxemics the scientific understanding of the amount of space people feel they need between themselves and others.

salpingo refers to the fallopian tubes, which are the small tubes connected to the uterus from the ovaries, by which means the eggs produced by the ovaries travel to the uterus, as part of the menstrual cycle.

stammer the involuntary pausing and the repeating of the initial letters of a word or words. This is similarly referred to as a stutter; although to stammer is the more polite term to describe the difficulty the person has in getting words out fluently.

References

ACT Academic (2018) Online library of Quality, Service Improvement and Redesign tools. SBAR communication tools: situation, background, assessment, recommendation. *NHS Improvement*. Available at: https://improvement.nhs.uk/documents/2162/sbar-communication-tool.pdf (accessed 29 July 2020).

Ali, M. (2017) Communication skills 2: overcoming barriers to effective communication. *Nursing Times*, 114(1): 40–42. Available at: www.nursingtimes.net/clinical-archive/assessment-skills/communication-skills-2-overcoming-the-barriers-to-effective-communication-18-12-2017/ (accessed 18 January 2021).

Ali, M. (2018) Communication skills 6: difficult and challenging conversation. *Nursing Times*, 114(4): 51–53.

Allen G.P., Moore W.M., Moser L.R., Neill K.K., Sambamoorthi U. and Bell H.S. (2016) The role of servant leadership and transformational leadership in academic pharmacy. *American Journal of Pharmaceutical Education*, 80(7): 113. doi: 10.5688/ajpe807113.

Alzhrani, F. (2019) Objective and subjective results of the Bonebridge transcutaneous active direct-drive bone conduction hearing implant. *Saudi Medical Journal*, 40(8): 797–801. Available at: www.ncbi.nlm.nih.gov/pmc/articles/PMC6718859/ (accessed 20 August 2021).

Axtell, R.E. (1998) *Gestures: The Do's and Taboos of Body Language around the World*, 2nd ed. University of Michigan: Wiley.

Baile, W.F., Buckman, R., Lenzi, R., Glober, G., Beale, E.A. and Kudelka, A.P. (2000) 'SPIKES' – A six-step protocol for delivering bad news: application to the patient with cancer. *Oncologist*, 5: 302–311. Available at: https://theoncologist.onlinelibrary.wiley.com/doi/full/10.1634/theoncologist.5-4-302 (accessed 21st February 2021).

Ballantyne, H. (2017) Undertaking effective handovers in a healthcare setting. *Nursing Standard*. Available at: https://journals.rcni.com/nursing-standard/undertaking-effective-handovers-in-the-healthcare-setting-aop-ns.2017.e10598 (accessed 20 July 2020).

Barrow, J.M. and Sharma, S. (2021) Five rights of nursing delegation. *StatPearls*. Available at: www.ncbi.nlm.nih.gov/books/NBK519519/ (accessed 2 November 2021).

Bass, C. and Halligan, P. (2014) Factitious disorders and malingering: challenges for clinical assessment and management. *Lancet, 19*; 383(9926): 1422–1432. Available at: www.thelancet.com/journals/lancet/article/PIIS0140-6736(13)62186-8/fulltext (accessed 19 January 2021).

Beamish, A.J., Foster, J.J., Edwards, H. and Olbers, T. (2019) What's in a smile? A review of the benefits of the clinician's smile. *Postgraduate Medical Journal*, 95: 91–95.

Becker, M.H. (1974) The health belief model and sick role behaviour. *Health Education Monographs*, 2(4): 409–419. Available at: www-jstor-org.proxy.library.lincoln.ac.uk/stable/45240625?seq=1#metadata_info_tab_contents (accessed 31 January 2022).

Berwick, D. (2013) *A Promise to Learn – A Commitment to Act. Improving Patient Safety in England. National Advisory Group on the Safety of Patients in England.* Available at: https://assets.publishing.service.gov.uk/government/uploads/system/uploads/attachment_data/file/226703/Berwick_Report.pdf (accessed 21 January 2021).

Black, A.L. and Curtis, J.R. (2002) Communicating bad news. *Western Journal of Medicine,* 176(3): 177–180. Available at: www.ncbi.nlm.nih.gov/pmc/articles/PMC1071708/ (accessed 19 August 2021).

Bogdashina, O. (2014) Top 5 Autism Tips: Managing Sensory Overload. Available at: www.autism.org.uk/advice-and-guidance/professional-practice/sensory-differences (accessed 20 August 2021).

British Medical Association (BMA) (2020) 2020/21 General Medical Services (GMS) Contract Quality and Outcomes Framework (QOF) Guidance for GMS Contract 2020/21 in England. Available at: www.england.nhs.uk/wp-content/uploads/2020/09/C0713-202021-General-Medical-Services-GMS-contract-Quality-and-Outcomes-Framework-QOF-Guidance.pdf (accessed 25 October 2021).

British Tinnitus Association (2021) What is tinnitus? Available at: www.tinnitus.org.uk/what-is-tinnitus (accessed 20 August 2021).

Bushman, B.J. and Anderson, C.A. (2001) Is it time to pull the plug on hostile versus instrumental aggression dichotomy? *Psychological Review,* 108(1): 273–279.

Bussard, M.E. and Lawrence, N. (2019) Role modelling to teach communication and professionalism in prelicensure nursing students. *Teaching and Learning in Nursing,* 14(3): 219–223.

Caplan, M. (2014) *Touch Is to Live: The Need for Genuine Affection in an Impersonal World.* Chino Valley: Hohm Press.

Collini, A., Parker, H. and Oliver, A. (2021) Training for difficult conversations and breaking bad news over the phone in the emergency department. *Emergency Medical Journal,* 38(2): 151–154. doi: 10.1136/emermed-2020-210141.

Crew, B. and Levins, A. (2019) The prison as a reinventive institution. *Theoretical Criminology.* Available at: https://journals.sagepub.com/doi/full/10.1177/136248061984 1900?casa_token=JQWPRC-8FqsAAAAA%3AgGyOfPe_WXIBOjJ4vp8YqlG-D3Ocpn7 6JiRPO10I1hL4tQzaSDo89svzALHRwkGjqejgReDtoFEx4A (accessed 19 January 2021).

Dang, S. (2015) Six ways measles can affect the eyes. *American Academy of Ophthalmology.* Available at: www.aao.org/eye-health/tips-prevention/six-ways-measles-can-affect-eyes-2 (accessed 24 August 2021).

Department of Health and Social Care (2018) Stronger Protection from Violence for NHS Staff. Available at: www.gov.uk/government/news/stronger-protection-from-violence-for-nhs-staff (accessed 22 February 2021).

Dowding, D. and Thompson, C. (2004) Using decision trees to aid decision making in nursing. *Nursing Times,* 100(21): 36. Available at: www.nursingtimes.net/roles/nurse-managers/using-decision-trees-to-aid-decision-making-in-nursing-25-05-2004/ (accessed 26 September 2021).

Dunning, D. and Kruger, J. (1999) Unskilled and unaware of it: how difficulties in recognizing one's own incompetence lead to inflated self-assessments. *Journal of Personality and Social Psychology,* 77(6): 1121–1134. Available at: CiteSeerX 10.1.1.64.2655. doi: 10.1037/0022–3514.77.6.1121. PMID 10626367 (accessed 5 November 2021).

Ekman, P. (2003) *Emotions Revealed*, 2nd ed. New York: Times Books.

Entwistle, F. (2013) Francis in brief: key nursing recommendations. *Nursing Times*. Available at: https://cdn.ps.emap.com/wp-content/uploads/sites/3/2011/05/Francis-report-3.pdf (accessed 29 November 2020).

Eunson, B.I. (2015) *Communicating in the 21st Century*, 4th ed. Queensland: John Wiley and Sons.

Foss, C. (2002) Gender bias in nursing care? Gender-related differences in patients' satisfaction with the quality of nursing care. *Scandinavian Journal of Caring Sciences*, 16(1): 19–26. Available at: https://pubmed.ncbi.nlm.nih.gov/11985745/ (accessed 18 August 2021).

Frank, A.W. (2012) From sick role to practice of health and illness. *Medical Education*, 47(1): 18–25.

Frank, M.G. (2001) Facial expressions. *International Encyclopedia of the Social and Behavioral Sciences*. Oxford: Elsevier, pp. 5230–5234.

Glambek, M., Skogstad, A. and Einarsen, S. (2017) Workplace bullying, the development of job insecurity and the role of laissez-faire leadership: a two-wave moderated mediation study. *International Journal of Work, Health and Organisations*, 32(3). Available at: www.tandfonline.com/doi/full/10.1080/02678373.2018.1427815 (accessed 2 November 2021).

Gogate, P., Gilbert, C. and Zin, A. (2011) Severe visual impairment and blindness in infants: Causes and opportunities for control. *Middle East African Journal of Ophthalmology*, 18(2): 109–114. Available at: www.ncbi.nlm.nih.gov/pmc/articles/PMC3119278/ (accessed 24 August 2021).

Hall, E.T. (1977) *Beyond Culture*. New York: Doubleday.

Hall, C., Stubbs, J. and Dickens, G. (2014) *Verbal Orders: Are You Up to Date with Current Guidance?* Available at: www.researchgate.net/publication/264325021_Verbal_orders_are_you_up_to_date_with_current_guidance (accessed 15 July 2020).

Harwood, R.H. (2017) How to deal with violent and aggressive patients in acute medical settings. *Journal of the Royal College of Physicians: Edinburgh*, 47: 176–182.

Health Education England (2016) *Make Every Contact Count (MECC): Consensus Statement*. Available at: www.england.nhs.uk/wp-content/uploads/2016/04/making-every-contact-count.pdf (accessed 26 September 2021).

Health and Safety Executive (HSE) (1996) *Violence at Work: A Guide for Employers*. UK: HSE.

Hefzy, E.M., Wegden, A.A. and Abdel Wahed, W.Y. (2016) Hospital outpatient clinics as a potential hazard for healthcare associated infections. *Journal of Infection and Public Health*, 9(1): 88–97. Available at: https://pubmed.ncbi.nlm.nih.gov/26264392/ (accessed 10 March 2022).

Hess, D.R. (2005) Facilitating speech in the patient with a tracheostomy. *Respiratory Care*, 50(4): 519–525.

Higgins, J., Wilson, S., Bridge, P. and Cooke, M.W. (2001) Communication difficulties during 999 ambulance calls: observational study. *British Medical Journal*, 323(7316):

781–782. Available at: www.ncbi.nlm.nih.gov/pmc/articles/PMC57355/ (accessed 19 January 2021).

Hinduja, S. and Patchin, J.W. (2009) *Bullying Beyond the Schoolyard: Preventing and Responding to Cyberbullying.* Thousand Oaks, CA: Corwin Press.

HM Prison and Probation Service (2019) *Prison Drug Strategy.* Available at: https:// assets.publishing.service.gov.uk/government/uploads/system/uploads/attachment_ data/file/792125/prison-drugs-strategy.pdf (accessed 19 January 2021).

HMSO (2005) *Mental Capacity Act.* Available at: www.legislation.gov.uk/ukpga/2005/9/ contents/enacted (accessed 21 February 2021).

HMSO (2010) *Equality Act.* Available at: www.legislation.gov.uk/ukpga/2010/15/ contents (accessed 18 August 2021).

HMSO (1983) *Mental Health Act.* Available at: www.legislation.gov.uk/ukpga/1983/20/ contents. (accessed 21 February 2021).

HMSO (2018) *General Data Protection Regulations.* Available at: www.gov.uk/ government/publications/guide-to-the-general-data-protection-regulation (accessed 21 July 2020).

Höglander, J., Eklund, J.H., Spreeuwenberg, P., Eide, H., Sundler, A.J., Roter, D. and Holmström, I.K. (2020) Exploring patient-centred aspects of home care communication: a cross-sectional study. *BMC Nursing,* 19(91). doi: https://doi.org/10.1186/s12912-020-00483-1.

Jack, K., Hamshire, C. and Chambers, A. (2017) The influence of role models in undergraduate nurse education. *Journal of Clinical Nursing,* 26(23–24): 4707–4715.

Johnson, K.L. (1988) The touch of persuasion. *Broker World,* April.

Kaufman, E. (2017) How Patients experience the Trauma Bay: surprising findings from patient interviews. *Leonard Davis Institute of Health Economics.* Available at: https://ldi.upenn.edu/ healthpolicysense/how-patients-experience-trauma-bay (accessed 19 January 2021).

Kawabata, T., Ohbuchi, K., Gurieva, S., Dmitrieva, V., Mikhalyuk, O. and Odintsova, V. (2016) Effects of inexpressive aggression on depression in college students: cross cultural study between Japan and Russia. *Psychology,* 7: 1575–1586. doi: http://dx.doi. org/10.4236/psych.2016.713152.

Kenaszchuk, C., Reeves, S., Nicholas, D. and Zwarenstein, M. (2010) Validity and reliability of a multiple-group measurement scale for interprofessional collaboration. *BMC Health Services Research,* 10(83). doi: http://dx.doi.org/10.1186/1472-6963-10-83.

Kjellmer, G. (2009) Where do we backchannel? On the use of mm, mhm, uh huh and such like. *International Journal of Corpus Linguistics,* 14(1): 81–112.

Krug, E.G, Dahlberg, L.L., Mercy, J.A., Zwi, A.B. and Lazano, R. (eds.) (2002) *World Report on Violence and Health.* Geneva: World Health Organisation.

Kübler-Ross, E. (1969) *On Death and Dying: What the Dying Have to Teach Doctors, Nurses, Clergy and Their Own Families.* New York: Scribner.

Lamotte, G., Shouman, K. and Benarroch, E. E. (2021) Stress and central autonomic network. *Autonomic Neuroscience: Basic and Clinical,* 235. doi: 10.1016/j.autneu.2021.102870. Available at: https://search-ebscohost-com.proxy.library.lincoln.ac.uk/login.aspx?dir ect=true&db=edselp&AN=S1566070221001004&site=eds-live&scope=site (Accessed 31 January 2022).

Lawton, S. and Carol, D. (2005) Communication skills and district nurses: examples in palliative care. *British Journal of Community Nursing*, 10(3). Available at: www-magonlinelibrary-com.proxy.library.lincoln.ac.uk/doi/pdf/10.12968/bjcn.2005.10.3.17619 (accessed 8 February 2021).

Levitt, D.H. (2001) Active listening and counsellor self-efficacy: emphasis on one microskill in the beginning counsellor training. *The Clinical Supervisor*, 20(2): 101–115. doi: 10.1300/J001v20n02_09. S2CID 145368181.

Lowry, M. and Lingard, G. (2016) Deescalating anger: a new model for practice. *Nursing Times*, 112(4): 4–7.

Luft, J. and Ingham, H. (1955) 'The Johari window, a graphic model of interpersonal awareness', Proceedings of the western training laboratory in group development. Los Angeles: UCLA.

Makaton.org (undated) *How Makaton Works*. Available at: www.makaton.org/TMC/About_Makaton/How_Makaton_Works.aspx (accessed 24 August 2021).

Martin, G., Ghafur, S., Cingolani, I., Symons, J., King, D. and Arora, S. (2019) The effects and preventability of 2627 patients' safety incidents related to health information technology failure: a retrospective analysis of 10 years of incident reporting in England and Wales. *The Lancet*. Available at: www.thelancet.com/journals/landig/article/PIIS2589-7500(19)30057-3/fulltext (accessed 28 November 2020).

Martinez, L. (2019) *A Professional's Guide to Sensory Impairment. The OT Practice: Experts in Therapy*. Available at: www.theotpractice.co.uk/news/our-experts-blog/a-professional-s-guide-to-sensory-impairment (accessed 20 August 2021).

Matsumoto, D. and Hwang, H.S. (2011) *Reading Facial Expressions of Emotion*. Available at: www.apa.org/science/about/psa/2011/05/facial-expressions (accessed 31 July 2020).

McColm, R., Brown, J. and Anderson, J. (2006) Nursing intervention for the management of patients with mania. *Nursing Standard*, 20(14): 46–49.

McKinnon, J. (2016) *Reflection for Nursing Life: Principles, Process and Practice*. Oxon: Routledge.

Mcquail, D. and Windhall, S. (2015). *Communication Models for the Study of Mass Communications*. London: Routledge.

Meehan, T.C. (2001) Therapeutic touch as a nursing intervention. *Journal of Advanced Nursing*. Available at: https://doi.org/10.1046/j.1365-2648.1998.00771.x (accessed 19 June 2020).

Mehrabian, A. (1972) *Non-verbal Communication*. New Jersey: Transaction Publishers.

Morris, D. (2002) *Peoplewatching: The Desmond Morris Guide to Body Language*. London: Vintage.

Moule, P., Armoogum, J. and Taylor, J. (2017) Evaluation and its importance for nursing practice. *Nursing Standard*, 31(35): 55–63. Available at: https://journals.rcni.com/nursing-standard/evaluation-and-its-importance-for-nursing-practice-ns.2017.e10782#:~:text=Evaluation%20is%20important%20in%20healthcare,how%20well%20something%20is%20working.&text=Nurses%20are%20well%20placed%20to,base%2-0for%20effective%20care%20delivery (accessed 24 September 2021).

Murphy, T. (2001) *The Angry Child: Regaining Control When Your Child Is Out of Control.* New York, NY: Three Rivers Press.

Narayanan, V., Bista, B. and Koshy, C. (2010) 'BREAKS' protocol for breaking bad news. *Indian Journal of Palliative Care,* 16(2): 61–65. Available at: www.ncbi.nlm.nih.gov/pmc/articles/PMC3144432/ (accessed 21 February 2021).

National Institute for Health and Care Excellence (NICE) (2015) *Costing Statement: Violence and Aggression. Implementing the NICE Guidelines on Violence and Aggression (NG10).* Manchester, UK: National Institute for Health and Care Excellence.

National Institute for Health and Care Excellence (NICE) (2020) *Scenario: Acute Epistaxis.* Available at: https://cks.nice.org.uk/topics/epistaxis-nosebleeds/management/acute-epistaxis/ (accessed 26 September 2021).

National Institute for Health and Care Excellence (NICE) (2021a) *Shared Decision Making.* Available at: www.nice.org.uk/about/what-we-do/our-programmes/nice-guidance/nice-guidelines/shared-decision-making (accessed 10 March 2022).

National Institute for Health and Care Excellence (NICE) (2021b) *Standards Framework for Shared Decision Making, Support Tools, Including Patient Decision Aids.* Available at: www.nice.org.uk/corporate/ecd8/chapter/background-and-context#patient-decision-aids (accessed 26 September 2021).

National Patient Safety Agency, General Medical Council and British Medical Association (2004) *Safe Handover: Safe Patients. Guidance on Clinical Handover for Clinicians and Managers.* London: British Medical Association.

Navarro, C.D., Castelao, E.L., Hadfields, A., Pierce, S. and Szyld, D. (2021) Clinical debriefing: TALK to learn and improve together in healthcare environments. *Trends in Anaesthesia and Critical Care,* 40: 4–8. Available at: www.sciencedirect.com/science/article/pii/S2210844021001052 (accessed 19 January 2021).

Neades, B. (2013) Aggression. In: Dolan, B. and Holt, L. (eds.) *Accident and Emergency Theory into Practice.* London: Bailliere Tindall, pp. 183–189.

NHS (2018) *Blindness and Vision Loss.* Available at: www.nhs.uk/conditions/vision-loss/ (accessed 31 January 2022).

NHS Choices (2019) *Symptoms – Bipolar Disorder.* Available at: www.nhs.uk/mental-health/conditions/bipolar-disorder/symptoms/ (accessed 19 August 2021).

NHS Digital (2020) *Cervical Screening Programme, England 2019–2020.* Available at: https://digital.nhs.uk/data-and-information/publications/statistical/cervical-screening-annual/england---2019-20 (accessed 25 October 2021).

NHS England (2012) *Introducing the 6Cs.* Available at: https://www.england.nhs.uk/6cs/wp-content/uploads/sites/25/2015/03/introducing-the-6cs.pdf (accessed 9 March 2022).

NHS England (2013) *Compassion in Practice – One Year On.* Available at: www.england.nhs.uk/wp-content/uploads/2016/05/cip-one-year-on.pdf (accessed 20 January 2021).

NHS Leadership Academy (2013) *Healthcare Leadership Model.* Available at: www.leadershipacademy.nhs.uk/wp-content/uploads/2014/10/NHSLeadership-LeadershipModel-colour.pdf (accessed 31 January 2022).

NHS Resolution (2019) *Being Fair: Supporting a Just and Learning Culture for Staff and Patients Following Incidents in the NHS*. Available at: https://resolution.nhs.uk/wp-content/uploads/2019/07/NHS-Resolution-Being-Fair-Report-2.pdf (accessed 2 June 2021).

Nibblelink, C.W. and Brewer, B.B. (2018) Decision-making in nursing practice: an integrative literature review. *Journal of Clinical Nursing*, 27(5–6): 917–928. Available at: https://pubmed.ncbi.nlm.nih.gov/29098746/ (accessed 10 March 2022).

Nursing and Midwifery Council (NMC) (2010) *Guidance on Using Social Media Responsibly*. Available at: www.nmc.org.uk/globalassets/sitedocuments/nmc-publications/social-media-guidance.pdf (accessed 11 July 2020).

Nursing and Midwifery Council (NMC) (2018a) *The Code: Professional Standards of Practice and Behaviour for Nurses, Midwives and Nursing Associates*. Available at: www.nmc.org.uk/standards/code/#:~:text=It%20is%20structured%20around%20four,and%20promote%20professionalism%20and%20trust (accessed 30 July 2020).

Nursing and Midwifery Council (NMC) (2018b) *Delegation and Accountability. Supplementary Information to the NMC Code*. Available at: www.nmc.org.uk/globalassets/sitedocuments/nmc-publications/delegation-and-accountability-supplementary-information-to-the-nmc-code.pdf (accessed 5 November 2021).

Nursing and Midwifery Council (NMC) (2018c) *Standards of Proficiency for Registered Nursing Associates*. Available at: www.nmc.org.uk/standards/standards-for-nursing-associates/standards-of-proficiency-for-nursing-associates/ (accessed 28 August 2021).

O'Daniel, M. and Rosenstein, A.H. (2008) Professional communication and team communication. In: Hughes, R. (ed.) *Patient Safety and Quality: An Evidence Based Handbook for Nurses* (Volume 1). Maryland: AHRQ, pp. 271–284.

Oberai, H. and Anand, I.M. (2018) Unconscious bias: thinking without thinking. *Human Resource Management International Digest Journal*, 26(6): 14–17.

Omer, R., Patel, S. and Soloman, D. (2020) Covid-19 and Ethnicity: How the Information Gap Exacerbates Inequality. *The BMJ Opinion*. Available at: https://blogs.bmj.com/bmj/2020/10/08/covid-19-and-ethnicity-how-the-information-gap-exacerbates-inequality/ (accessed 18 August 2021).

Osborne, H. (2012) Making social media work professionally. *The Guardian*, 8 June 2012.

Owen, P. (2018) Leading by example: if nurses can think about how to be exemplary role models, we can teach the next generation leadership skills without trying. *Primary Healthcare*, 28(5): 14.

Palmer, M.J., Clarke, L., Ploubidis, G.B. and Wellings, K. (2019) Prevalence and correlates of 'sexual competence' at first heterosexual intercourse among young people in Britain. *British Journal of Medicine: Sexual Reproductive Health*, 45: 127–137. Available at: https://srh.bmj.com/content/familyplanning/45/2/127.full.pdf (accessed 18 August 2021).

Pearce, L. (2018) How to make handovers more effective. *Nursing Standard*. Available at: https://rcni.com/nursing-standard/features/how-to-make-handovers-more-effective-141126 (accessed 27 July 2020).

Pham, H., Puckett, Y. and Dissanaike, S. (2017) Faster on-scene times associated with decreased mortality in Helicopter Emergency Medical Services (HEMS) transported trauma patients. *Trauma Surgery and Acute Care Open*, 2(1). Available at: www.ncbi. nlm.nih.gov/pmc/articles/PMC5887760/ (accessed 19 January 2021).

Pieterse, A.H., Stigglebout, A.M. and Moouton, V.N. (2019) Shared decision making and the importance of time. *Journal of American Medical Association*, 322(1): 25–26.

Press Association (2009) Hospital staff suspended for playing Facebook 'lying down game'. *The Guardian*, 9 September 2009.

Price, O., Baker, J., Bee, P. and Lovell, K. (2015) Learning and performance outcomes of mental health staff training in de-escalation techniques for the management of violence and aggression. *British Journal of Psychiatry*, 206(6): 447–455. doi: 10.1192/bjp.bp.114.144576.

Rosenzweig, M.Q. (2012) Breaking bad news: a guide for effective and empathic communication. *Nurse Practitioner*, 12, 37(2): 1–4. Available at: www.ncbi.nlm.nih.gov/pmc/articles/PMC5578619/ (accessed 21 February 2021).

Royal College of Nursing (RCN) (2020a) Nurses are undervalued because they are mostly women, a new study finds. Available at: www.rcn.org.uk/news-and-events/news/uk-nurses-are-undervalued-because-they-are-mostly-women-new-study-finds-290120 (accessed 18 August 2021).

Royal College of Nursing (RCN) (2020b) Promoting patient safety. *RCNi*. Available at: https://rcni.com/hosted-content/rcn/first-steps/promoting-patient-safety (accessed 29 November 2020).

Royal College of Physicians (2017) *NEWS2: Standardising the Assessment of Acute-Illness Severity in the NHS*. London: Royal College of Physicians.

Royal National Institute for Deaf people (RNID) (2018) *Facts and Figures*. Available at: https://rnid.org.uk/about-us/research-and-policy/facts-and-figures/ (accessed 25 August 2021).

Royal Pharmaceutical Society (2019) *Professional Guidance on the Administration of Medicines*. Royal Pharmaceutical Society.

Schramm, W. (1954) How communication works. In: Schramm, W. (ed.) *Process and Effects of Mass Communication*. Illinois: University of Illinois Press, pp. 18–26.

Scottish Government (2011) Principles of Inclusive Communication: An Information and Self-Assessment Tool for Public Authorities. Available at: www.gov.scot/publications/principles-inclusive-communication-information-self-assessment-tool-public-authorities/pages/9/ (accessed 26 August 2021).

Social Care Institute for Excellence (SCIE) (2020) *Dignity in Care*. Available at: www.scie.org.uk/dignity/care/communication (accessed 19 January 2021).

Sooriyamoorthy, T. and De Jesus, O. (2021) Conductive Hearing Loss. In: *StatPearls*. Treasure Island, FL: StatPearls Publishing. Available at: www.ncbi.nlm.nih.gov/books/NBK563267/ (accessed 20 August 2021).

Sorokowska, A., Sorokowski, P., Hilpert, P., Cantarero, K., Frackowiak, T., Ahmadi, K., Alghraibeh, A., Aryeetey, R., Bertoni, A., Bettache, K., Blumen, S., Błażejewska, M., Soares Bortolini, T., Butovskaya, M., Castro, F., Cetinkaya, H., Cunha, D., David, D., David, O.,

Pierce, D. (2017) Preferred interpersonal distances: a global comparison. *Journal of Cross-Cultural Psychology*, 48. doi: 002202211769803.10.1177/0022022117698039.

Tanna, R.J., Lin, J.W. and De Jesus, O. (2021) Sensorineural hearing loss. In: *StatPearls*. Treasure Island, FL: StatPearls Publishing. Available at: www.ncbi.nlm.nih.gov/books/NBK565860/ (accessed 20 August 2021).

Thompson, C., Cullum, N. and McCaughan, D. (2004) Nurses, information use, and clinical decision making – the real world potential for evidence-based decisions in nursing. *Evidence-Based Nursing*, 7: 68–72.

Truman, C. (2019) I would like to give an idea of what a good nurse role model looks like. *Nursing Times*. Available at: www.nursingtimes.net/students/i-would-like-to-give-an-idea-of-what-a-good-nurse-role-model-looks-like-26-11-2019/ (accessed 1 September 2021).

Tucker, C.M., Marsiske, M., Rice, K.G., Jones, J.D. and Herman, K.D. (2011) Patient-centred culturally sensitive health care: model testing and refinement. *Health Psychology*, 30(3): 342–350. Available at: www.ncbi.nlm.nih.gov/pmc/articles/PMC3092156/ (accessed 18 August 2021).

UNICEF (2019) *Baby Friendly Standards*. Available at: www.unicef.org.uk/babyfriendly/about/standards/ (accessed 17 June 2020).

UK Prison Population Statistics (2020) Available at: https://commonslibrary.parliament.uk/research-briefings/sn04334/

Velentzas, J. and Broni, G. (2014) Communication cycle: definition, process, models and examples. In: *Recent Advances in Financial Planning and Product Development*. WSEAS Press, pp. 177–131.

World Health Organisation (WHO) (1992) The ICD 10 Classifications of Mental and Behavioural Disorders. Geneva: WHO.

World Health Organisation (WHO) (2010) Telemedicine: opportunities and developments in member states. Report on the second global survey on ehealth. *Global Observatory for Ehealth*, 2. Switzerland: WHO. Available at: www.who.int/goe/publications/goe_telemedicine_2010.pdf

World Health Organisation (WHO) (2013) *Blindness and Vision Impairment: Refractive Errors*. Available at: www.who.int/news-room/q-a-detail/blindness-and-vision-impairment-refractive-errors (accessed 25 August 2021).

World Health Organisation (WHO) (2020) *Human Papillomavirus (HPV) and cervical cancer. Fact Sheet*. Available at: www.who.int/news-room/fact-sheets/detail/human-papillomavirus-(hpv)-and-cervical-cancer (accessed 18 August 2021).

Image credits

Figure 1.2: www.communicationtheory.org/shannon-and-weaver-model-of-communication/

Figure 1.4: www.researchgate.net/publication/311739283_A_Multimodal_Nonverbal_Human-Robot_Communication_System

Figure 1.5: www.communicationtheory.org/riley-riley-model-of-communication/

Index